NOW, WHERE DID I PUT MY GLASSES?

NOW, WHERE DID I PUT MY GLASSES?

Caring for Your Parents – A Practical and Emotional Lifeline

Jackie Highe

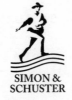

**SIMON &
SCHUSTER**

London · New York · Sydney · Toronto

First published in Great Britain by Simon & Schuster UK Ltd, 2007
A CBS COMPANY

3 5 7 9 10 8 6 4

Simon & Schuster UK Ltd
1st Floor
222 Gray's Inn Road
London WC1X 8HB

www.simonandschuster.co.uk

Simon & Schuster Australia
Sydney

A CIP catalogue for this book is available
from the British Library.

ISBN 978-0-7432-9531-4

Typeset in Times by M Rules
Printed and bound in the UK by
CPI Mackays, Chatham ME5 8TD

This book is dedicated to the memory of my parents,
Jack and Lily Barraclough, and my parents-in-law,
Phil and Nancy Highe

CONTENTS

ACKNOWLEDGEMENTS

I want to thank Sheena Scriven, friend and wonderful community staff nurse; Sue Beavers, one of the best care home matrons in Britain; the doctors, health care workers, funeral directors, coroner's officers and other professionals right across the UK, who allowed me into their worlds.

Thank you too to all the marvellous charities and organizations that do so much to support the elderly and their families: in particular Help the Aged, Age Concern, the Alzheimer's Society and Carers UK, for their knowledge and helpfulness.

But above all I'm grateful to the generous people who told me their stories and shared their feelings with such complete candour. Without them there would be no book.

INTRODUCTION

We don't want it to happen, they don't want it to happen, but sooner or later it happens all the same – our parents grow old. It's a huge responsibility for families. How can you all come through it with grace, keeping their dignity intact along with your sanity – and everyone's sense of humour?

This book will help you to do that. It will take you inside people's personal experiences; give you insights from everyone's point of view. Elderly parents will tell you in their own words what they thought and felt when their doctor – and their children – were saying they couldn't live at home any more, and children tell you how they felt about saying it; there are family stories on everything from home helps to hospitals, from selling their house to power of attorney – and death. It's a long list and it takes you on a journey that begins before any problems appear.

It's a practical guide too, unravelling the labyrinths of the NHS, social services, care homes, and all the other organizations you might have to deal with; it will walk you through the financial and legal complexities you'll encounter.

The voices in this book will help you deal with what's happening in your own life. They're moving, perspective-changing, sometimes funny – and strangely cheering; they're the voices of people who know; they've been there, felt the guilt, faced the fear, torn their hair, agonized over decisions. Everyone's experience is different but – as this book will show you – you're not alone.

Chapter 1

TALKING TO EACH OTHER

'When I get old, just put me to sleep.'

Many of us say this, or something like it, usually when we're in our prime and have no concept of what it means, or feels like, to grow old – old age is so far away and unreal as to be unimaginable.

It seems that built into our survival mechanism is the feeling we'll live forever. We're the only species on the planet to be consciously, intellectually, aware that we'll age and die, yet somehow that knowledge doesn't carry any conviction. We're able to blot it out; it happens to other people, not us. It's essential for the human spirit to sideline it or we could waste our whole lives in anxiety and fear, incapacitated by the anticipation of old age and death.

The older we get the more we cling to what makes life good for us, and as the years go by we tend to think even less about what might be ahead – after all, there's plenty of time yet. And it's true – there *is* more time. In 1901 the life expectancy of women was 49, and for men it was just 45. So our comparatively recent ancestors were lucky if they made it to 60. If they did they'd probably feel and look ancient and suffer from a variety of complaints that modern medicine and technology have done an enormous amount to alleviate, even

1

eradicate. We're living longer and in a healthier state than ever before. There's a good chance we'll still be feeling young and looking good at 70, and many of us will live well into our eighties and nineties.

It's wonderful. But it's also dangerous, because it lulls us into a false sense of security. There's no need to think about getting old. Often the first realization that *we* aren't immortal comes when we start to realize our parents aren't. But even that feeling wears off – your parents went through it with their own parents but they'll have got over it by now and probably won't be ready to think about their own age yet.

So no one talks about it – the subject isn't brought up. Questions, the answers to which could change lives profoundly for better or worse, remain unasked. Questions like: What do you expect/want to happen if you get to the stage where you can't look after yourself? Have you made a will? If you ever start to become mentally frail will you be prepared to give one of us power of attorney? And even – do you want to be buried or cremated?

It's hard enough to broach subjects like these if you're fortunate enough to be part of a close, loving family; if you don't get on with your parents or siblings, if your parents are estranged, divorced, remarried, or you simply all live a long way apart, then it can seem impossible.

But it's important you talk about the future while it *is* still the future and ageing issues are still unthreatening. Otherwise you could suddenly find yourselves in the middle of a crisis with no clue as to what to do next, no idea what your parent/s would want – or what *you* want – and forced to make big decisions quickly when you're under a lot of stress.

The Communication Gap

One of the acknowledged major factors in the breakdown of relationships is that we don't talk to each other. The result can be a complete failure to understand what's going on in the other person's head. We get aggressive, defensive and angry; we cast blame, make excuses and accusations. We're thinking about *our* position, only seeing our own point of view. It's not necessarily selfish – the other person is doing exactly the same thing.

This lack of understanding can apply particularly between elderly parents and their children when it comes to issues of ageing. Because it's such an emotive subject it tends to produce kneejerk reactions on both sides.

Half the battle is in understanding what your parents are feeling, and the other half is in understanding what *you're* feeling – and then talking to each other about those feelings.

From your point of view you're looking ahead, trying to be sensible. You're thinking: 'It's for their own good. I'm only trying to help, and this is all the thanks I get. Why are they being so awkward? Don't they realize that planning now will mean they can do things *their* way, and they'll be able to keep control for longer. They don't understand how the law works. I've tried to explain but they don't seem to get it.'

Things will look very different from your parents' point of view. Just try to imagine what it feels like to be in their place – think yourself into it. They're very possibly going to be in denial – if they don't anticipate old age then it won't happen. And it's admitting weakness, that there might come a time when they won't be master of their own destiny. It doesn't bear thinking about – so they don't think about it. (When our turn

3

comes we'll probably feel exactly the same.) They might resent the fact that *you* seem to be thinking about it, and may worry about your reasons. 'Do they think I'm losing it? Do they want to take over?' And however you look at it, it's an invasion of their privacy, involving money issues and other intensely personal aspects of their lives. 'It's my business, not theirs. Why are they patronizing me? Do they think I'm stupid?'

So both sides can have entrenched – and, when you look at it, equally justifiable – points of view. Families will be thinking of the practical angle without perhaps imagining how hard it must be for anyone to be pragmatic about the fact that they'll eventually die. Parents themselves could just see it as interference and not credit their children with the simple desire to help.

Laura got into exactly that position with her mother Annie, who is 72 and lives in the same town. They've both tried to take the high ground and the result is an impasse.

'Why are they nagging me about a will? I'm not telling them how much I'm worth if that's what they're after' – Annie, aged 72

Laura says:

'Mum's always been the argumentative type and I've got a temper, so sometimes we've fallen out, though never for long. My two brothers both live miles away and they don't really get involved.

'Dad's been dead for eight years and now Mum's living with a man who's divorced and got kids and grandchildren of his own. We don't like him much, to be honest, and my brothers got on to me and said we ought to get the will question sorted out. They're worried because she's bought a house with him and it could get complicated.

'They won't admit it, but I think they're afraid her step-family will get her money, rather than us. Of course, they said as I lived nearer and saw her more often it was *my* job to bring it up.

'So one day I mentioned to her that we were wondering if she'd made a will. She went completely ballistic. She told me to mind my own business; it was her money to do what she liked with. We had a really dreadful row. I wasn't being nosy and Mum should have known me better than that. It upset me so much I didn't speak to her for weeks.

'She came round eventually and we're back on speaking terms, although I'm not sure she trusts me like she did before, which hurts. And we still don't know if she's made a will. I can see it being a real hassle when she dies. And what happens if she gets Alzheimer's or something? I wish now I'd led up to it more gently. I suppose I can see why she jumped down my throat – it must have looked cheeky, me blurting it like that, but I was nervous!'

Annie probably knows, deep down, that she ought to make a will, but she doesn't want to face it, which is making her prickly. She might be worried about how to leave what she has, or maybe she's already made up her mind and suspects that what she's decided will cause arguments between the two sides of her family – a family that already seems to have tensions. Those will feel like very good reasons for letting things drift.

But she might have lashed out because she's feeling guilty about it. If Laura, instead of getting angry too, had taken a breath and said why she was worried – because there could be a legal mess – the fight might have been avoided.

Laura needs to tackle her mother again when the dust has settled, and try to explain this time. She could say something like, 'You know, Mum, we really weren't trying to pry, but if you don't have a will things could get complicated. You don't have to tell us what's in it or make any of us executors if you don't want to . . .'

By understanding what's *really* worrying your parents you can address those worries more effectively, talk to them about their concerns. It's important too to express your own anxieties – explain properly, don't be afraid to show your weaknesses. If they know they're not the only ones with something to be vulnerable about, they won't feel so insecure.

Conversations like this can help you all realize nothing is black and white, everyone has insecurities, and there could be room for manoeuvre – maybe that there's nothing to fight about at all.

Getting It into the Open

You may have such a relaxed relationship with your parents that you can come right out and say: 'Look, Dad, I know you're only 72 and in good shape, but I was thinking . . . now's the time to start telling me what you want me to do when you get old.' But for many people that's as impossible as a walk on Mars.

In fact, millions of families habitually don't talk at all about their emotions. Everyone's so busy it can be rare to sit down together for a meal – when would they find the time to bare their souls?

Andy's father Fred is 72. He and Andy's mother divorced twenty-five years ago and he remarried and had a second family of his own, as well as bringing up his second wife's children.

'Mum's living with a chap and has a share in their house, but I haven't asked her about the future. I suppose I would if she started sliding downhill. I'd want to protect her. Dad's quite well off but we've no idea what his plans are. I don't know how to bring it up. He's always liked being in control – to lose it would kill him. You see people torn apart by this. My brother isn't bothered and there doesn't seem to be any rush, so we've left it alone.

'The trouble is, we're rarely all together just as a family, there are always other people there – my dad's wife, my half-sisters and stepsisters – so it's difficult to talk about really personal things.'

But there are ways of bringing up these touchy subjects without it seeming as though you can't wait for your parents to die. The first thing is to be casual, not make a big deal out of it. Rather like the first time you try to have the big sex chat with your child, if you sit them down solemnly and say, 'We need to have a talk,' the warning flags will go up.

Trevor's 78-year-old father Clive seemed unapproachable.

'Although Dad's quite tough for his age, I know he's not as fit as he was, but I was frankly afraid of bringing up the future. He's got a terrible temper and I absolutely didn't want to have a fight. But then there was a story line on one of the soaps about a man with an extended family who had all kinds of fallings out, will problems and so on. On the Sunday lunch-time Dad and I had popped out for a beer and I just asked him if he'd seen it – I knew he was a fan. It wasn't planned but we got on to how you see families torn apart, talking about what we'd have done in their place, as you do with the soaps.

'We started having a real discussion – there was no pressure because it was just about a TV show – and I found he had views I'd never have guessed.'

7

'Listening to him I was surprised – underneath he was much softer than the independent type I knew. We didn't come to any conclusions or make any decisions. It stayed hypothetical – we never got down to brass tacks. But I think we'll be able to talk about it again now, maybe make some plans. I feel much better about the whole thing, and I think it will have made him ask himself some questions.'

Whether they spring from a story on TV, in the newspapers, or whether a relative or neighbour is going through something relevant, events can open the door for a chat. It's gossip, it's about someone else, it's safe.

You'll all have an opinion. If yours is different from your parents', say so and say why, just as you would if you were chatting about a more innocuous subject, but don't rubbish their ideas or argue, even if you think they're wrong. Instead listen and get a feel for what they're thinking.

Try to have a laugh too. At the end of a conversation like this you can say, 'Seriously, is that what you'd really like, because eventually we'll have to deal with it and we want to get it right.' The response might include, 'I'm not dead yet!' but you'll have broken the ice and paved the way for the subject to be brought up again later.

But what if that doesn't happen? What if you can't even get that far?

Jenny's parents, Sid and Marjorie, are in their early seventies and live a couple of hours away from her. They're still reasonably fit, but she can see their health isn't as good as it was and she's worried.

'They totally ignore the idea of being old. I can't even broach the subject – and I hate to think how they'll cope.'

'Dad's used to having everything his own way and Mum running round after him. She even carries his pills about to dole out. He regards that, and the cooking and cleaning and so on, as women's work. And Mum only knows how to care for him. They're very much products of their generation. Whichever one goes first, the other just won't be able to handle it, physically or psychologically.

'Dad can't cook at all and he's diabetic. If Mum died he'd eat all the wrong things – junk food and fish and chips – and it would kill him. Mum would manage better, but then again I'm afraid she'd just give up. Her life revolves round Dad and if he died her reason for living would be gone.

'We need to talk about it all because we live so far away. I work very long hours and my husband's job covers weekends, so we have to make a big effort to see them every few weeks. My brother's family live nearer, but he and his wife both work full time and they've got kids.

'Dad got in a mess with the video and he called my brother then fell out with him because he couldn't get there straight away. He doesn't seem to understand that you can't always just drop everything and come running.

'We know they've made wills because they've told us they're saving their money for us all to inherit. We keep telling them to spend it, but they can't seem to do it. It goes against a lifetime of being careful. And it will cause problems down the line, because I know when the time comes they won't want to spend it on things like home care or anything to make their lives easier.

'I'm sure Dad just assumes that when they get older everyone will rally round and nothing much will change for them, but I know it isn't going to be like that – it's physically impossible.'

Maybe Jenny could turn her father's rather prewar attitude to women into an opening. She knows that although he takes Marjorie for granted he loves her deeply, and she could use this as a reason for starting to think and plan for the future. 'What would happen to Mum if you died? Do you think we should talk about it, Dad?'

Keep Talking

Even if your parents seem unapproachable the most important thing of all is to keep talking – on any and every subject. Keep the lines of communication open. Families who get used to exchanging feelings and sharing emotions will find it easier to talk about this most fraught of topics when the time does come.

If you've tried to bring it up and been fobbed off or even shouted at, don't take the bait and let a rift develop – be flexible. If you don't fall out about it you can always try again later.

Attitudes change – you never know ... a subject that causes hackles to rise this year could be brought up by your parents themselves next year.

This happened with Mavis. She's 84 and lives in Scotland. Her son Lachlan and his family are in the south of England.

'She's a fantastic lady, really young at heart, and has always led a pretty full life, but when Dad died three years ago we thought it was a good time to bring up the future. After all, at over 80 she isn't going to be this sprightly forever and we're hundreds of miles away. We're her only family, although she does have a lot of friends in Scotland – she's lived there all her life.

'We suggested she move nearer to us so that as she got older we'd be well placed to organize things for her, look after her and so on. It cut no ice at all. She said she didn't need our help – which in fact was true at the time – and she "wasn't ready to be scooped up and transplanted" or even to talk about "getting old". We had to leave it there.

'Then a few months later she phoned us and said, "OK, family conference, up you come" – so we did. She told us her eyesight was deteriorating and she'd discovered she might lose her sight. She was amazing. She'd been thinking about what we said and, although she had no intention of moving to England, she was ready to discuss the future.

'We had a good talk about what she needed at that point and what she'd prefer to happen down the line if her eyesight was worse and she got to the stage where she couldn't look after herself.

'We arranged some privately paid-for cleaning help in the house immediately, and we've been able to think ahead and make some enquiries for the future, so if anything happens suddenly we know where to look for the right help straight away. She's been involved in everything.

'She's told us exactly what she wants us to do. It's great because we can talk to her about it any time. She's interested in the whole subject now and it's become a family joke – "when I get old".'

Lachlan and his family were concerned about Mavis but they didn't try to push her into moving south. Instead they were patient and let it lie for a while. Because of this she felt safe to open the subject again when her circumstances changed – she wasn't afraid she'd be bullied into anything.

When you do manage to get a dialogue going it's worth remembering that what your parents say now and what they might say later could change, especially about things like where they'll live. It's one thing to speculate about going into a home, sheltered housing, living with you and so on, when it all may never happen – it could be another thing altogether when it comes to the crunch (see Chapter 4). But it won't have been wasted – you'll all have a basis to start from. And if you've kept the subject open you'll be likely to understand why they've changed their minds.

Talk amongst Yourselves

It's important you talk to partners, siblings and other members of the family, not just your parents. You need to know each other's views. Younger siblings might be expecting the eldest to take a parent to live with them, for example, or that the one with the biggest house should do it. You might find your parents are confidently expecting to live with a particular member of the family, and this may or may not be what that person wants or can manage.

Jo made this discovery. Her mother Alice is a 79-year-old widow who has no other children.

'When we brought it up Mum was quite happy to talk about the future. She just said, "Well, I'm going to be living with you, aren't I?" She'd just assumed it.'

'We said it wouldn't be possible because there's not enough room and nowhere to build a granny flat, even if we could have afforded it. It upset her at first but when we explained it wasn't that we didn't love her, but that we physically couldn't do it, she started thinking about her options. It was a good job we discussed it early because we'd had no idea she was taking it for granted.'

It would have been devastating for Alice to find this out at the point when she was having to come to terms with giving up her own home. Although she was disappointed she couldn't live with her daughter, at least she had time to look at other possibilities with her, and to keep control of her future.

Surprises can be pretty hard on partners too, as Don's wife Sue found out. His father Mel is a very fit 80-year-old.

'I want Dad to live with us when the time comes. I couldn't put him in a home. I haven't spoken to him about it but I'm sure it's what he'll want too. I hadn't mentioned it to Sue, either. We had my grandma to live with us when I was a kid, so it seemed natural.

'Then it cropped up one day at home and Sue went mad. She said there's no way she's going to take all that on. She works full time and has parents of her own – what would *they* think? Was I expecting her to look after them all? I never thought she'd feel like that. It's a good job I haven't mentioned it to Dad – I might easily have done.'

Don's situation shows how vital it is to talk about how *you* feel. Getting a clear idea of what everyone thinks before you bring it up with your parents might save a lot of heartache – and rows – later.

It's not just the issue of care; it's questions like who'll be executors to a will, who'll take the enduring power of attorney. These are potentially rich seams of resentment, jealousy and family rifts unless they're addressed at an early stage. The guides below will help get you past the first hurdle.

Guide 1 – Some Questions to Raise

- **Have you made a will?**
  They don't need to tell you what's in it – but it's best to make one straight away. Point out that you've made yours (you should have!). See Chapter 7.
- **Would you be prepared to give one of us enduring power of attorney?**
  You don't use it until/unless necessary. See guides in Chapter 7.
- **What would you want to do if you had to give up your home?**
  Emphasize there are no decisions to be made about anything. If they say they want to live with family, then talk over what it would mean. See Chapter 4.
- **Do you want to be buried or cremated? And in church or not?**
  If their spouse has already died, do they want to be treated in the same way when they die? Probably the best way to raise this tricky subject in the first place is to make a light comment, just to get the ball rolling.

Guide 2 – When Having a Conversation

Do

- Keep it light-hearted and relaxed – reassure them
- Ask what they think and why – and really listen to the answers
- Be honest – say what you think and feel, and why
- Discuss *all* possibilities, not just your ideas and theirs
- Involve the rest of the family – know what *you'd* all prefer too
- Be objective – don't take things personally
- Remind them you love them

14

Don't

- Lose your temper or have a row
- Push your views
- Break off communication
- Produce any leaflets on anything in advance – they might feel railroaded

Guide 3 – Understanding Each Other

What parents say	What they might mean
I'm not old	I don't want to be old
I don't need a will – I'm not dying	If I make a will it means I'm going to die
There's plenty of time	I don't like thinking about it
It's not your business	I'm still in control
I don't need your help	Do you think I'm senile?
I can manage	I can't bear not to manage – I'm afraid

What you say	What they think you mean
Are you OK?	You're not OK
Let us help with that	You can't do it yourself
This is how it works	You can't keep up – you're past it
You're not as young as you were	You're living on borrowed time
You need to make a will	What are you leaving me?
Will you take out power of attorney?	We want to take over

At a Glance

- Try to start talking while it's still hypothetical
- Discuss with your partner/siblings, etc. too
- Put yourself in your parents' place
- Be prepared to do research – but as a follow-up, not in advance

Chapter 2

WHEN THEY START TO NEED SOME HELP

We take our parents' existence for granted. They've always been there – older, more grown-up than us – and we tend to imagine they always will be. Whatever their role in our lives, however big or small a part they play, they make us feel young. They're a visible, living token that *we* aren't old.

Families split, arguments break out, sides are taken, people lose touch, remarry – but despite the turbulent dynamics of Third Millennium family life our parents are our roots. They've cared for us, made decisions on our behalf and given advice (asked and unasked). Whatever we achieve in our lives, to them we'll always be the children they brought into the world. Whether we like it or not, whether we like *them* or not, whether they live together or apart, they retain a proprietorial interest in us that comes from having conceived us in the first place.

So when it starts to dawn on us that our respective roles are beginning to reverse, it's a seismic shift in our universe, hard to grasp and even harder to accept. To think that our parents are becoming our responsibility instead of the other way round makes us uncomfortable, sad. We don't want to watch them lose their independence; we don't want to be the ones to take it away.

It's worse for them. Imagine if someone said to you today, sorry, but your freedom, your choices, your control – everything that makes your life *yours* – is about to start sliding into the sunset because you're no longer capable of living your life completely unassisted. Would you be happy to sit back and let it happen?

Of course, giving up your independence isn't an overnight event. Often it's a slow, insidious process, a gentle chipping away, a little bit of help here, a bit more there; but it's inexorable – and frightening. No wonder people resist taking even the very first steps on this road; it can feel like the beginning of the end.

But appropriate help as soon as it starts to be needed, even if it's only a small amount, can lengthen the time your parents remain independent, and increase their comfort, security, happiness and quality of life not just physically, but by giving them – and you – peace of mind, and freedom from worry and stress.

Spotting the Signs

It's not easy to tell when problems first start to develop, partly because none of you wants to believe it's happening and partly because changes can be so slight neither you nor they might notice. This is especially true if you see a lot of your parents. They might be getting a little less physically active, have more trouble bending down or reaching up, but how do you quantify that? Their eyesight or hearing or short-term memory might be deteriorating – but very slowly.

If you live a long way away or don't visit them very often you might notice a step change, but you could easily ignore the signs, and your parents are almost certain to push them aside – after all, they'll tell themselves, even 20-year-olds have the occasional senior moment.

'I don't need a home help – that's for old people' – Eileen, aged 89

On the other hand they could be telling you everything's OK and suppressing the fact they're struggling because they 'don't want to be a burden'. They might even be afraid that somehow they'll be slapped into a care home against their will.

In fact, social services and doctors are keen to help the elderly stay in their own homes because it's believed they'll be happier, healthier and more active both mentally and physically if they maintain as much control as possible over their lives. All the many services and care packages available are specifically aimed at making it possible for them to do this (see the guides at the end of this chapter and Chapter 3).

So if they don't ask for help, how do you tell? Look out for signs of tiredness or even exhaustion. Do they seem a bit down? Watch to see if the house starts looking a little neglected. Is the kitchen or bathroom a bit dirtier than you'd expect? Are their clothes as clean as usual?

Do they seem to be losing weight? Not bothering to make proper meals can be an indication they're struggling. Have a quiet look at what's in their kitchen cupboards and fridge when you're making a cup of tea. Is there enough food in the house – are they eating well or starting to cut corners? If you think they might be, ask them casually what they had for lunch/dinner.

Chat about food in a relaxed and general way and you may find they volunteer that they don't bother to cook as much as they used to. Then you can ask why. Take the same relaxed approach to other things – housework, getting up the stairs, shopping – so they're more likely to confide in you. If you sweep in and try to organize them they could bristle and accuse you of interfering. They'll be feeling defensive – anyone would – and the last thing you want is a row.

None of these things means your parents are physically incapable or falling apart mentally, but all or any of them could be a hint they need some extra help to cope.

Couples

If both your parents are still alive and living together, they'll probably be able to manage at home for longer than singles because they'll help each other, sharing chores and each taking on the jobs they do best. But at the same time that can make it very hard to spot when they do need help unless they tell you – and they might not.

One partner might start to fail before the other, who could try to cope just as they've always coped, telling themselves it's not serious, it's a blip, everything is all right. They can hide things from you (and from health visitors and doctors) for a surprisingly long time this way without necessarily meaning to – just through not wanting to make a fuss.

'I can't keep running to you; jobs need doing' – Helen, aged 82

Alan's parents, Ron and Helen, are both in their eighties. Helen has angina, while Ron is almost blind and his short-term memory is beginning to go, but for a long time they were active, went for walks, did the shopping, cleaned the house and cooked. Alan and his brother both live several hours' drive away.

'They always sounded cheerful on the phone – my mother was even perky – but when they came to stay for a couple of weeks she had one or two weeps and told my wife that nobody knew what she had to do for my dad. We dug a bit and found that, fiercely independent and angry with himself at not being able to do things, he was making life hard for her in lots of ways.

'My parents belong to a time when the man was the head of the family and the woman took care of him. Dad had always run the finances, done the household repairs. Mum had never learned to drive.

'She wouldn't accept any help and insisted on taking up more and more of his slack – at one point she even donned a boiler suit and climbed a ladder with a sieve over her face to spray a wasps' nest in the eaves! She told us about it with great hilarity and pride and we all smiled, even though we quailed at the thought of her up a ladder.

'We told her she had sons to do that for her, and she said, "I can manage. I'll tell you when I can't" – but of course she never did. We'd tackle all the jobs when we went to stay, and I fitted a grab rail over the bath, but the only other help they'd agree to was someone to tidy up the garden every couple of weeks. We couldn't force them – we were trying to let them live *their* way. Then suddenly Mum had some kind of seizure and went into hospital.

'She fought back from the brink of death but her personality seemed to have changed completely. From cheerful, practical and down-to-earth she became, almost overnight, bitter, resentful, irrational, accusing us of conspiring against her – wild things. She told us the hospital was out to get her and imagined all kinds of dreadful scenarios. This inoffensive little old lady suddenly started shouting and attacking the nurses. We were worried to death.

'We were told that personality changes like this aren't uncommon. Psychiatrists were called in and gradually it became clear that the stress of looking after Dad on her own had been wearing her down. On the outside she'd been coping, but bottling up the worry, combined with her unsuspected illness, had given her a kind of nervous breakdown. She recovered but she's much frailer – her health is permanently damaged.

'I'd say to anyone with elderly parents, don't take what they say about how they're getting on at face value, even when they seem fine.'

'Try to dig deeper, even if they insist everything's OK. We thought we were watching carefully, but we still didn't see how far she was stretched. She hid it because she didn't know how to let go.'

Alan's experience highlights how difficult it can be to get at the truth. Your parents might not actually lie to you but they're likely to put the most favourable interpretation on things because that's how they see it themselves.

Singles

In theory it can be easier to spot the warning signs when a parent is living alone – there's no one to cover for them. What's more, doctors and social services should be aware they're alone, although you can't rely on this – if they've been in reasonable health they may not have seen a doctor or health visitor for a while.

It has to be said that GPs, like social services, vary; some are more proactive than others. It isn't really safe to assume someone else is taking notice.

Raj is 20 and at college. He visits his 78-year-old grandmother Annapuma when he goes to stay with his father. Annapuma has been widowed for five years and lives in her own house.

'I stay with Dad every three or four months and always pop in to see Gran. When I lived with Dad I didn't bother to go much but when I started college he said I might come back one day and she'd be dead, so I make a bit more effort now.

'Gran's great – she sits me down, makes me eat loads of food and we have a good chat. When I leave she pushes a bar of chocolate into my hand. I think she must save them for me in the drawer for ages because they always taste stale, but I never tell her so!'

'Then I went round one day and I was shocked at the state of the house – I mean, I'm not that particular but even I could tell it needed a good clean. Gran wasn't looking all that well either.'

'I didn't like to say anything to her myself so I mentioned it to Dad, but he isn't good at noticing that sort of thing – he's not much on housework himself. He said it was Gran's business but I twisted his arm and he went round to have a chat with her about it. It turned out she'd had a fall, got badly bruised and not told anyone because she didn't want anyone to think she was past it, so she was struggling on.

'Dad insisted she saw the doctor and then both of them talked her into having some help cleaning the house, getting into the bath, and so on. They told her it could be temporary and when she got better she could stop it if she liked.'

Raj spotted the change in his grandmother because he hadn't seen her for a while. His father, who saw her every week, didn't notice anything until it was pointed out to him.

If you live a long way from your parents, it's worth alerting social services and asking them to keep an eye open. Things can go downhill quite quickly.

Giving up Driving

This is one of the hardest things to do and it's easy to see why. It's a big milestone – once you give up your car you lose your freedom of movement and instantly become dependent on lifts and public transport. You're grounded.

If your parents live right in a town centre where facilities are within walking distance they might manage, but there are still the shopping bags to carry, the steep hill to negotiate on foot and so on. If they live almost anywhere else, without a car it will be impossible to lead the life they led before. Routine trips to the doctor, optician, supermarket can be exhausting.

What was simple – a visit to the garden centre, meeting friends, a pub lunch, choir practice – becomes complicated, involving taxis or phoning round, constantly asking favours. They don't like to do that – who would? So their social life shrinks.

Eloise is 90 and had to give up her car when her eyesight failed.

'I do get rather lonely now I can't go out under my own steam. My daughter and her husband come down about once a month but hardly ever with my grandchildren, who are off on gap years and things. I only see my sister once a year because she lives so far away.

'My friends are dying one by one. I miss them. If my husband were alive I'd have more of a social life – people don't ask you round when you're on your own. I watch a lot of TV. Just seeing one other person makes a difference.'

Elderly people in Eloise's position are bound to feel isolated when they stop driving. They can become almost reclusive, and this might lead to depression. Lifts to a day centre a couple of days a week could transform their lives.

If your parents belong to a club or group of any kind it's

quite likely their fellow members will give a hand, especially if they're members of a church. And local voluntary groups do hospital outpatient runs. You'll find them in the front of the phone book, in the parish magazine, and social services will have a list.

George is 82. He gave up driving at 80, although reluctantly, because although they live near the shops, his wife Jean has osteoporosis and can't walk very well.

'It was on my family's mind and they'd mentioned it a few times but I'd hung on to the car because I didn't want my wife to be housebound. I was driving into the next town and suddenly realized I just didn't want to go – I was afraid of tackling the traffic. Roundabouts and dual carriageways were beginning to scare me – my reactions were getting slower.

'Then one day I cut a corner really badly and my son-in-law saw me do it! He made no bones about it. He told me it was just the sort of thing he was worried about and I couldn't really disagree. Still, we discussed it for months – it wasn't an instant decision.

'I regret it but I'm living with it, and you know, it's only been two years but if I were to get behind the wheel now, I don't think I'd be able to drive.

'It's saved us so much money. We can afford to take the odd taxi. Our travelling days are not quite over – we're content.'

Public transport can be patchy and unreliable but your parents might feel it's extravagant to take a taxi, so it's worth reminding them just how expensive a car is to maintain. Giving it up will release cash they'll be glad to spend on other things without feeling guilty.

But with so much at stake it's no wonder your parents will

hang on to their car for as long as possible – and very probably longer than they should for their own and everyone else's safety. For men, too, it can be a loss of masculinity.

Mathew's father Henry was still driving at 88.

'He had a huge estate car which he'd been driving for years, and would never swap it for something smaller. He said it would do for him, but I think he was nervous about having to learn how to drive something different, which at his age is more than understandable. But it was much too big for him. He's so tiny he couldn't see straight through the windscreen – he was looking through the top half of the steering wheel at the road.

'When he came to see us we'd watch him turning into the drive with our hearts in our mouths. He regularly took the corner too wide and swung over the lawn. In fact we dug up a conifer to give him a clear run in. Whenever he left I'd try to see him out, but he'd reverse down our drive, straight out into the road and, very often, right across the street on to our neighbour's lawn – mercifully we live at the end of a very narrow, quiet cul-de-sac. When our neighbour pointed out to him that he was on her grass he told her, "Well, you know, I can't see." She was very good about it! Of course it couldn't go on – he was going to kill himself, or someone else. But he wouldn't budge.

'We asked his local bobby to go and have a quiet word with him and point out that he wasn't just risking his own life. It worked, because he agreed straight away, where we'd been trying for years to persuade him.'

It's always going to be hard to persuade your parents to give up driving. You can't force them; they can just ignore you, which is what Henry had been doing to Mathew. That's why he decided to bring in someone from outside – he knew a policeman is an authority figure that someone of Henry's generation would respect.

It's a scary thought but sometimes a near miss can be the

breakthrough that changes their minds. Sarah is a 94-year-old widow whose eyesight is deteriorating. She lives in a tiny village and her car was literally a lifeline.

'My niece had told me it was time to stop driving, as had several friends, but I couldn't imagine how I'd manage. There's no shop in the village, no doctor – no anything really. I had to keep the car, I thought, to survive. One day I was at a road junction, looked both ways and pulled out. I'd thought it was clear but something was coming – I just hadn't seen it. I didn't hit it but I knew then my driving days were numbered.

'Word must have got around because my doctor came to see me. She sat down next to me, put her hand on my knee and said, "Have you considered giving it up?" Well, I know I'm getting on, so I didn't put up any resistance. It's terribly restricting though. People are kind but you can't always be asking for lifts, especially at night. I do get the bus to the supermarket sometimes.

'You hope people will say, "I'm just going to Tesco, do you want anything?" but they don't. So you feel bad about ringing them up to ask for a separate trip.'

Arranging Help

At first, the only help your parents need may be as simple and informal as a weekly lift to the supermarket, or someone to do their shopping for them, pick up prescriptions and so on. Maybe they'd appreciate a hand with the vacuuming, laundry or tidying the garden.

You could also offer to stock their freezer with ready-meals to reheat on days when they don't feel like cooking. If you do this, try to take them shopping with you so they can choose for themselves. It might be tempting – and easier – to supply them with a selection you think they'll like and will be good for them, but who'd want to lose control of something as fundamental as food?

Family, friends and neighbours might be able to cover all this between you without involving any outside agencies, but it's worthwhile fixing up a regular arrangement. Your parents won't like to keep asking, and if it becomes routine – 'on Thursday Sue always takes us to Sainsbury's' – then they'll feel they're being less of a nuisance.

It's good to spread the load among several people for backup and to prevent anyone feeling put upon – something that can very easily happen. People lead busy lives and, especially among families, resentment can grow amazingly quickly if one or two people feel they're taking all the strain.

If your parents need some help in the house, again it can be possible to do it between you – but they might take some persuading.

'I'm not having any stranger cleaning under *my* beds' – Jane, aged 93

Mary's mother-in-law Jane was a robust 93, a redoubtable lady with a will of iron. She lived just down the road and Mary's husband Bob would pop in every evening on his way home from work. Most days Mary would drop by for a cup of tea and a chat and to give her a hand. She'd often take some dinner for her too.

'Jane was very agile for her age and took pride in still doing her own housework. I did her washing and ironing and Bob would tackle any odd jobs that needed doing. She still used to moan we didn't do enough!

'Her daughter lives just a few miles away, but she just let us do it all. I have to say that was something I found a bit wearing. We were the nearest, it's true, but I think she used it as an excuse to do nothing.

'When we tried to persuade Jane to have some proper help she was adamant. She was horrified at the idea of having a stranger "rummaging about" in her cupboards. It wasn't an easy house to look after either – it had a steep flight of stairs up to the bedrooms and we were always worried she'd pitch herself down them. She looked after herself right until her last illness, when she went into hospital.

'I wish now we'd involved her GP more. He might have been able to persuade her where we failed, and she'd have been entitled to all kinds of assistance, although the idea of what she called "charity" appalled her. But we should have persevered – as much for our sake as for hers. It was a constant, huge worry, a lot of work, and the responsibility wore us down.'

'I'm not sorry we did it for her, but my own mother is getting frailer now and I'm not going to take on all that again. We've talked about it and I think – I hope – she'll be reasonable, but you never know.'

If there's no one to help you and/or you live far away, it can be too much of a strain to maintain this level of care. But before you get any kind of assistance from the local authority they'll first want to assess your parents.

Where to start

The best way to start is either to talk to social services, or your parents' GP, and they'll send a social worker to look at their circumstances, health, and physical and mental capabilities – everything from their ability to do the shopping and cooking to getting in and out of the bath.

In England and Scotland this should all happen from one assessment, while in Wales and Northern Ireland the various departments might have to be approached separately for their own assessments.

They'll talk to your parents (you can be there) and ask them how they're managing, what they can/can't do. It can feel intrusive but they won't get any help without it. Then a care manager will outline what help your parents should get and who will provide it – help could come direct from social services or the NHS, but some of it may be contracted out to private companies or charities.

What services they'll qualify for will depend entirely on their local authority – they all have their own rules and criteria – but once they've assessed your parents as having certain needs, they have to provide for them (although not necessarily for free). Your parents are entitled to a copy of this assessment, and have the right to query it if they don't agree with its findings.

Of course, if you or your parents are planning to pay for any help yourselves you can just go ahead – social services will have a list of companies who offer all kinds of services. But it's worth having an assessment anyway because you'll get the benefit of professional advice on what's needed, and learn about what's on offer – and there's a lot. Some volunteer agencies/charities provide free services. You can contact them directly but they might ask for a social services' referral, which will need an assessment.

In either case you might find they have to wait for the assessment, depending on how efficient the local authority is, social services' workload, and how urgent they think it is. Your parents can't insist on a time limit, although they can complain if they think they've waited too long.

When it comes to paying for care at home, England, Northern Ireland, Scotland and Wales all have different rules and, on top of that, every local authority has its own policy. In England and Wales they'll means-test your parents and decide whether they need to contribute towards their care, and if so, how much. In Scotland some types of care are free to over-65s and in Northern Ireland some care is free to over-75s (see the guides at the end of Chapter 3).

Charlotte is 90 and lives alone. Her daughter Angela lives about forty miles away and persuaded her to have help with cooking and cleaning, which Charlotte pays for.

'It wasn't easy to persuade her at first. She insisted she was fine, but we'd visit and there would be stuff everywhere because she couldn't see to pick it up. And she was living on snacks – she's never been much of a cook anyway. Then I mentioned how much pleasanter it would be for her to have someone else doing the work – as I said to her, *I've* got a cleaner. I pointed out that we weren't trying to take over; she could pay for it herself. It made her realize she's still in con-trol and she changed her mind.'

Charlotte herself is pretty relaxed about it. She lives alone so, as she sees it, her quality of life is in her own hands.

'I keep saying to myself, I'm old – I've accepted it. You have to adapt.'

'My brother-in-law can't walk well and refuses to have a stick. My poor sister chases after him. It's just vanity. You come to terms with age. I get to the bottom of the stairs and forget what I was going up for. My cleaner comes in a couple of times a week. She's marvellous and keeps me organized. She takes me shopping in her car. I have an alarm too. If I knock into it accidentally a voice comes on, asking me if I'm all right!

'I can't see well enough to cook so social services offered to deliver a hot meal every day. I gave way but they never brought lunch before two p.m. I told them I couldn't wait that long but they said I was at the end of the run. In any case I didn't think much of the food, so they gave me a leaflet about a company that delivers prepared frozen meals for me to reheat in the oven. They're much tastier and I can eat them when *I* want – but I have to pay a bit more for them than I did for meals on wheels.'

Charlotte has found a way to keep her independence but get enough support to keep her comfortable. She's fortunate she can afford to make her own choices. Social services won't usually provide cleaning on its own; there needs to be some element of personal care involved too – assistance with bathing, dressing, etc. Since Charlotte doesn't need this kind of help she wouldn't have been able to get any house-cleaning from her particular local authority. There are infinite variations on who pays for what, but it's fair to say almost everyone has to pay for something.

James and Peggy are 81 and 82. They live in a rented bungalow and a cleaner comes in once a week, which they pay for with the attendance allowance they claim (see the guides at the end of Chapter 3). Peggy needs some personal care because she has severe arthritis and can't reach up to cupboards or stand for too long, although she still cooks. James runs the vacuum round and they share the ironing. By doing everything in easy stages they manage well. Peggy can't walk far but she has a buggy and they do their own weekly shopping locally.

Peggy says:

'We have a marvellous family and we only have to pick up the phone, but we don't ask them for help unless it's imperative – we don't want to be a nuisance. We talked to our children about all this a few years ago when my arthritis started getting bad. We knew we wouldn't be able to manage indefinitely, so we faced facts and put our pride in our pockets.

'James can still keep the garden tidy but I wonder how long

that will last. I suppose eventually we'll just have to get someone in to do it. We've seen so many people go downhill. I hate
to think of it happening to us but we know it will – why pretend? I can't do what I did five years ago.'

And James says:

**'I wonder how many people of my age think deeply
about the future. I'm glad we can't see what's ahead – I
dread it. It's constantly on my mind but I try not to let it
get me down.'**

James and Peggy have accepted the reality, even though they
haven't much liked admitting they need help. What's more,
they're prepared to take more support if or when it becomes
necessary. The result is they're comfortable, relaxed and getting a lot out of life.

There's no doubt that arranging help is a complicated business. Basically, the system is there, and in theory your parents
should be able to get everything they need. In practice it
depends on how good their local authority is at dealing with
the elderly. Some areas are marvellous, others not so good.
The following guides should help you negotiate the maze –
just don't give up!

Guide 1 – Services

This is not an exhaustive list – local authorities and the NHS vary widely in what they can/will provide, and some areas have a wealth of charities and local voluntary organisations, while others aren't so well furnished. However, it will give you an idea of the breadth of services and help on offer and where to start looking.

Requirement	Social Services	NHS	Private Firms	Voluntary Organizations
Personal care once a day or more – help with bathing, getting in and out of bed, shaving, dressing, going to the toilet, meals, shopping, night care, etc.	They may contract some of this out to private firms and/or charities. (Varies across the UK.)		You can pay privately. Get an approved list and advice from Social Services or the UK Home Care Association. (See Guide 2 for contacts.)	Look in front of phone book, in your parish magazine or local papers. Social Services should be able to supply a list.
Daily hot meal delivery	May use Women's Royal Voluntary Service (WRVS).			WRVS
Weekly frozen meal delivery	Contracted out to private firms.		Social Services have a list.	
Home adaptation – wheelchair ramps, shower installation, stair rails, hand rails, etc.	Work under a maximum amount carried out free.		Citizens' Advice Bureaux (CAB) or Home Improvement Agencies. (See chapter 3.)	

Requirement	Social Services	NHS	Private Firms	Voluntary Organizations
Equipment – bath/shower raised toilet seats, etc.	Occupational therapist will assess.		CAB can give advice on companies supplying these items, or look in local phone book. (See Chapter 3.)	Disabled Living Foundation gives advice. (See chapter 3.)
Day centres/lunch clubs				Help the Aged or Age Concern (See Guide 2 for contacts.)
Mobility: wheelchairs, walking frames, sticks, buggies, etc.	Occupational therapist will assess.	Talk to GP about items available from the NHS	Social Services will have a list of companies.	The British Red Cross has an equipment loan service. (See Guide 2.)
Health Matters: occupational therapy, district nurse, chiropody, physiotherapy, etc.	Assessment	Talk to GP		
Home security: alarms, security equipment and fitting			Social Services will have a list of companies.	SeniorLink (a Help the Aged scheme – see Guide 2).

Guide 2 – Charities

There are national charities, voluntary organizations and agencies as well as local groups that offer help and/or advice. Take a look at the front of your phone book – you'll be amazed at how many there are. Here are just some of the main ones and how they can help. (There are more in Chapter 3.)

Organisation	What it Provides
Help The Aged Senior Line: 0808 8006565 Northern Ireland: 0808 8087575 To download leaflets: www.helptheaged.org.uk SeniorSafety: 01255 473999	Excellent free advice line for the elderly and their families. Free advice leaflets on many subjects. Phone for leaflets or ask Social Services. Also runs day-care centres in some areas. SeniorSafety Scheme offers security advice and some home fitting.
Citizens' Advice Bureaux Local phone number www.citizensadvice.org.uk www.adviceguide.org.uk	Free independent advice, face to face or on the phone. Leaflets on community care, benefits and much more.
UK Home Care Association 020 8288 5291 www.ukhca.co.uk	Information on private home-care companies who follow their code of practice.
Age Concern See local phone book for number	Day Centres, transport, home visits, shopping, information sheets.

Organisation	What it Provides
British Red Cross See local phone book for number www.redcross.org.uk	Drivers, loan of wheelchairs and medical equipment; some home care
Royal National Institute for the Deaf 0808 8080123 www.rnid.org.uk	Information on equipment
Royal National Institute for the Blind 0845 7669999 www.rnib.org.uk	Talking books, advice, some equipment
Volunteer Bureaux Volunteering England: 0845 3056979 www.volunteering.org.uk Northern Ireland Council for Voluntary Action: 02890 877777 www.nicva.org Volunteer Development Scotland: 01786 479593 www.vds.org.uk Wales Council For Voluntary Action: 0870 6071666 www.wcva.org.uk	Regional bureaux give information on services available locally. Volunteers make home visits, tidy the garden, do the shopping etc.
Counsel and Care 0845 3007585	Advice on how to choose a home-care agency
WRVS See local phone book for number	Hot meals, home visits, transport, shopping

At a Glance

- Look out for signs your parents are struggling
- Have a chat with them about help they might like
- Ask for a social services' assessment
- Look at what help is available through social services
- Check out local charities and voluntary organizations
- Ask social services for a list of approved private companies

Chapter 3

WHEN THEY NEED MORE CARE

As we go through life, whatever our mirror is telling us, inside our heads we're still young – our internal clock seems to stop for us at the point when we first felt truly grown-up. We know we're not that age any longer; we probably don't have the same opinions, maybe not even the same values, but we still feel we're essentially the same person – we're who we always used to be.

If that's true of us, it's just as true of our parents. They might have become used to making jokes about 'getting on a bit'. They'll say, 'I'm not as young as I was' – but they won't mean it.

The thing about old age is that it tends to creep up on us. We don't see it coming until suddenly there it is, right on our doorstep. We don't have time to adjust mentally to the reality because it's taken us by surprise. It's as though we wake up one morning to find the world has shifted on its axis overnight, and we don't occupy the same place in it any more.

This sounds rather dismal but in fact in some ways it's a good thing – there's a lot to be said for mind over matter. Not recognizing they're old can enable your parents to carry on independently for longer than if they sat and waited for old age to claim them. But there's a limit to how long they can do this, and a point where it can become dangerous to try.

If they do lose the ability to care for themselves without significant help it's still possible for them to live at home, but only if major changes take place – things like regular daily, even nightly, personal care, or maybe alterations to their house. And that means a change in everyone's attitude. They're not likely to welcome what they may see as an intrusion into their privacy, but the way you handle it can help them enormously in coming to terms with it.

There's a very long list of services and aids available, as they become increasingly disabled. Some are free, some not. It's sad to find it necessary but the right balance of care can keep your parents in their own home for far longer than you'd all have thought possible.

Keeping an Eye Open

If they've been getting on pretty well with a little bit of help you won't want to rock the boat. You'll be keen to let them get on with their lives, resisting the thought of more intrusive home care because you know they'll hate the idea and because it's another step nearer the end – and nobody wants to think about that.

But it's important to keep a close eye on them because at this stage changes can be serious. If your parents are already getting some help their social worker might spot things deteriorating, and their GP might notice if they're losing ground in eyesight and general health. He should certainly spot any changes for the worse if he's already treating them for serious complaints like diabetes, heart problems, arthritis and so on.

It doesn't always follow, though. GPs are busy – and although many are wonderful, some can be remarkably blasé. Gerry's mother Sheila is 82. She'd lived alone in her own bungalow since her husband died, and although she had high blood pressure she was taking medication for it.

'One day I got a call from the hospital saying that Mum had been admitted. She'd collapsed on the street and they suspected a broken hip. She was unconscious for two days and when they finally stabilized her sufficiently to do X-rays and other tests they found she hadn't broken any bones, but her sodium levels were dangerously low.

'Her GP told me that a loss of sodium wasn't uncommon in people who had been taking diuretics for years, as Mum had. He said he'd noticed a few months before that her level was dropping and had intended to test her again. She collapsed before he could do it.

'I'm not blaming her GP but I wonder why he didn't monitor her more frequently and keep it under control. Having very low sodium levels can be lethal – and in fact Mum almost did die.

'To be fair to the doctor, she hadn't been to see him about feeling unwell, but it had never been explained to her how important it was to watch this condition carefully. It should have been. If she'd realized she'd have gone for a checkup – Mum isn't a fool.'

Even the most conscientious doctors aren't mind readers, and elderly patients might not mention something that can turn out to be serious, particularly if it's left untreated. But there can sometimes be an alarming communication gap between professionals and the elderly they're dealing with. Not everyone finds it easy to relate to older people. What's more, our parents' generation was brought up to accept what doctors say at face value. It might not occur to them to ask for more detail.

It's worth trying to establish a relationship with your parents' GP, especially if you don't live nearby. Ask them to let you know if there's any change, and have a chat on the phone every now and then. They might not give you lots of private detail but at least they'll know to keep a careful watch, and who to phone in an emergency.

Ask your parents to tell you what medication they're on, what their doctor said at the last visit and so on. That way you'll have an idea of what to look out for too.

If you think they need more help, ask social services for an assessment (see Chapter 2). It won't matter if they've already been assessed; it can be done again because they're well aware that changes take place. At this stage the recommendations might involve personal care of an intimate kind, maybe frequent visits by a care worker more than once a day or at night, or possibly regular visits by a physiotherapist or other occupational therapist – it all depends on how they're coping.

The package may also suggest alterations to your parents' home. Doorways may need widening and ramps installing to accommodate a wheelchair; a downstairs bathroom may need fitting or a shower. The assessment might include equipment like a walking frame, a commode and other continence aids. Whatever they recommend, it's likely your parents will have to pay for at least some of it.

Small jobs that cost up to a maximum amount, like grab handles and extra banister rails, are usually provided free by the local authority without a means test. The drawback is they work to their own timetable, not your parents'. While there's no doubt they do jobs as quickly as they can, if they're busy it could mean a long wait.

Mike's father John is 84 and almost blind. When John's wife died, social services assessed him as needing various forms of care, including an extra banister rail.

Mike says:

'The local authority said they'd come in and do it, but weeks went by and still nobody turned up. We were worried Dad would fall down the stairs – he really couldn't see well at all. We live a long way away so one weekend I just took the stuff up there and fitted it myself. Luckily I could do the job otherwise I'd have paid someone to do it. A man from the council arrived a couple of months later and was quite surprised to find he wasn't needed.'

There's a complaints procedure. Don't hesitate to use it if you think things are going on too long. Your parents' safety and comfort are paramount.

For bigger jobs there are various grants and benefits, but they're not available to everyone. If your parents do qualify make sure any proposed work has been approved by whoever is paying for it before it's begun, or you could find payment being withheld.

Coming to Terms with It

It's one thing to have someone popping out for your prescriptions or doing your ironing – and quite another to accept the idea of a stranger coming in to help you do things like dress and undress. Your parents are understandably likely to resist any such suggestion as undignified and it can take a dramatic change in circumstances for them to come to terms with it.

Jill's in-laws, Will and May, were both 89 and, even though Will was almost blind, they'd been coping together until May broke her hip and went into hospital for several weeks.

'We knew Will wouldn't be able to cope for a minute on his own. We couldn't have him to stay with us because we're all out at work all day, and without May to keep an eye on him he'd have been a danger to himself.

'He was furious at the idea of an assessment but we explained that if he didn't have help he might have to go into a care home temporarily, and he hated the idea of that even more. What he wanted was to stay at home, and we were able to show him that this was the way to do it.

'Social services sent in a care worker three times a day. It was marvellous really, a huge weight off our minds. She'd help him out of bed, shower and get dressed, then do some cleaning, fetch his shopping and heat up a frozen lunch. She'd make sandwiches and leave them in the fridge for his tea, and someone would pop back later to help him into bed. He didn't need anyone in the night.

'He didn't much relish the thought of these women seeing him naked, but they were super ladies and we pointed out to him that they were only doing what the nurses had done when he'd been in hospital. That put a different slant on it for him.'

Finding a way to rationalize what can feel almost humiliating is important for your parents' pride, and as the threads of their life pass into other people's hands pride matters increasingly. Think how you'd feel . . .

In big and small ways it's enormously important to make an effort to save their dignity. Let them make their own decisions wherever possible. Try not to take over.

Rosalind's father Francis was left alone at 76 when his wife died. He lives at the opposite end of the country from Rosalind, but his son is only an hour away.

Rosalind says:

'Dad had always seemed fine. It never occurred to him to be old until Mum died. He'd had slight heart problems but they got worse and he was having trouble making the stairs. He doesn't make a fuss – you only know what he wants to tell you – but he took the initiative and talked to social services himself. He had a stair lift fitted and got a grant to help turn a downstairs room into a shower. They raised the sofa and bed for him too.

'He visits my brother once a week and my sister-in-law always sends him home with several pre-cooked meals to freeze. Now he has a couple of nice women coming in to give him a hand. He loves the attention. And why shouldn't he? He's entitled to have a fuss made of him.'

Rosalind stood back at first to give Francis time to realize for himself that he needed help, and as a result he's dealing with his altered lifestyle. He's got it under control and he's happy. If you don't feel you're in charge of your life, the opposite can happen.

Maggie is 87. She has one son who works on building contracts in Europe so she only sees him occasionally. She's diabetic, has severe osteoporosis and needs to spend most of her time in a wheelchair even to get around the house.

'When I got worse I struggled to get about, and there were days on end when I couldn't get out of bed. I'm ashamed to say I let myself get into a bit of a state.

'In the end my doctor made the moves. He sent social services round and they said I was going to be in a wheelchair and I'd need my doors widening, ramps putting in and other alterations. They did it, but it seemed to take ages and I was put into a local care home while the work was going on.

'Somehow nobody ever asked me what *I* wanted. They just seemed to take over. I could have argued, I suppose, but I knew it had to be done.'

'I've got carers coming in day and night to keep me going, and they mean to be kind, but sometimes they treat you as though you're not right in the head. I may be old but I'm not daft.'

Maggie has come up against something that's sadly not unusual. There can be a tendency to overpower elderly people who need help, especially on the part of professionals who are dealing with similar situations all the time. It's kindly meant, but a breezy 'we know what's best for you' approach is, if you think about it, rather insulting. After all, just the other day they were grown-ups able to make their own decisions and run their own lives without any help from an outsider young enough to be their child, or even their grandchild.

It's exhausting too – if you're a bit frail it won't take much to browbeat you into submission. You won't have the energy to put up a fight for long and in the end you might just give up and let it happen round you. Just think what it would be like if you had the flu and someone was pushing plans at you to redesign your kitchen.

As a family you can do a lot to counteract this by staying in touch yourself with social services and any other agencies involved. Talk to them regularly about what they're doing and why. Ask your parents how they're feeling about the care they're getting. Is it enough? Is it too much? Is there anything they'd change?

Approach everything calmly and give them time to think about things. Discuss alternatives if there are any. Wherever possible, allow them to choose for themselves and, above all, try not to fall into the trap of bullying with kindness.

Coping Day to Day

Your parents will be happiest if they can maintain a lifestyle as near as possible to the one they led before. The fact they've got help might be an enormous relief to you – and to your parents for that matter – but it comes at a high cost in self-esteem.

There are a lot of gadgets and aids available to help keep them independent and make their life easier and safer: everything from jar openers to spiky vegetable boards to special plug handles. The Disabled Living Foundation and Ricability both produce guides. Take your parents to visit the nearest Disabled Living Centre to try things out for themselves – even wheelchairs.

The more they can do for themselves the better they'll feel. Sam is a widower of 87 who has a daily care worker. His daughter Josie is proud of how he copes.

'Before Mum died Dad told her he'd look after the house – and he does. He uses one plate, one cup, one knife and fork, so there's never a lot of washing up to get on top of him, and he's developed his own routine. He finds things to fill his day.

'When he goes out he always changes into smart clothes. Otherwise, he says, he'd just turn into a slob. He does his paperwork, sorts his post and keeps track of bills. He spends time on his computer – he's just got broadband – and he's teaching himself the guitar.'

Sam's refusing to let life close down on him; he's prepared to tackle new things. As a result his horizons are still expanding and the days have some new excitement to offer. If you can suggest new hobbies and interests that might appeal to your parents, you'll be doing more than helping them enjoy themselves, you'll be keeping them attached to the world. They won't feel it's passing them by.

Marion's father Simon is 79 and has just fulfilled an ambition he's had for years but never found time for until now. She says: 'Dad's joined an art class and he's loving it. He says it's fantastic. The rest of the class is around Dad's age and the teacher is 84.'

The local library will have a list of evening classes, courses and clubs available in your parents' area. The University of the Third Age runs events and classes, including computer training. Encourage them to branch out – there are all kinds of bonuses. Apart from learning something they've always been interested in, honing a skill or talent, they'll meet a fresh set of people. It could give them a whole new lease of life.

Grandchildren and great-grandchildren can make a tremendous difference too. The more they can see of their grandparents, the better for them all. A special bond can form between the old and the young that enhances their lives. It keeps your parents in touch with the young world and it's marvellous for children because they'll get an insight into how earlier lives were lived, learn about their roots, and have precious memories that will be important to them as they get older themselves.

Michelle's grandmother Ada is 93 and lives several hours' drive away. She stays with Michelle a couple of times a year and loves to be around her teenage great-grandchildren.

Ada says:

'They're a bit loud round the house but I love them to bits. I can never work out what it is they're doing on those little computer things they carry around with them. They've tried to explain it but it goes beyond me. They come up and say, "Tell us about the war, Grandma Ada," and I'll talk to them about when I was a WAC. They seem to like it – they ask a lot of questions, and say, "We can't learn that at school." I've even helped them with their history projects.'

Ada needs quite a lot of personal care and so can only stay with her granddaughter for a few days a couple of times a year, when Michelle takes time off work to look after her, but she enjoys the bustle of family life. As she says, 'It makes a change and gives me something to look forward to.'

Michelle and Ada both know that to stay longer would be hard on everybody, but they haven't let the difficulty stop them from doing it altogether, because Ada gets such a kick out of it.

It can get beyond the point where visits like this are possible, though, as Brad and Hilary are finding. Brad's father Rick is 86 and lives 250 miles away.

'Dad always stays with us at Christmas and travels on the train now that he can't drive, but this year there were terrible delays and it took him nine hours to get here. He was freezing cold when we picked him up from the station and he stayed under the weather all through Christmas.

'My daughter's family always come too, but this year her boys really got Dad down. They're only two and four and we couldn't expect him to cope with them dashing round him, especially when he wasn't well. He loves to see them but he can't stand much. I think he'd like to take them out of a box and put them back when he's tired. They don't realize they're annoying him – they're just being kids. To the two-year-old he's just an old granddad and neither of them really knows him very well, which is a pity.'

Brad and Hilary know that Rick probably won't be strong enough to make it under his own steam another year. They're talking about going to fetch him next Christmas and taking him back afterwards, but this needs careful planning and maybe even time off work for one of them.

If he does come to stay they could try to set up a separate 'quiet room' where the children can leave their grandfather in peace for a while every day without him having to go out of the centre of things to his bedroom. Or they could tell the children that certain bits of the day are granddad's 'quiet times', when the living room is out of bounds for noisy games. He could maybe read them a story now and then, or watch a movie with them – relaxing activities they'll all enjoy.

If it's put to them that granddad gets a little bit tired because he's quite old, even small children can be very sympathetic and get into the spirit of things.

Keeping in Touch

Whether you live near your parents or not, it can be difficult to find time to visit them frequently. The weeks dash by so quickly. People are busier, working longer hours than ever before, and the prospect of spending a chunk of precious weekend in this way can, with the best will in the world, be unappealing (especially if you don't get on that well).

One of the saddest facts about family estrangement is that it can go on, sometimes with people not speaking to each other, until a parent dies, and then suddenly it's too late – you've lost the chance to tell them you love them. Many families who've found themselves in this situation say they'd give anything to turn back the clock.

Just dropping in for a cup of tea or sparing them a Saturday or Sunday now and then is going to show them they still matter to you. You have the power to light up their lives.

Phone calls can be a lifeline. A regular chat will keep them up to date with what's happening within the family, make them feel involved and help to keep them thinking about the world at large. Maureen phones her father Stewart, who's 90, once a week. He lives two hundred miles away and has a daily care worker.

'Dad loves our phone calls. He gets all steamed up about politics and enjoys a good discussion. It's our way of keeping tabs on him too because we can tell by the sound of his voice how he is.'

Sometimes, though, it can be hard to persuade them to chat. A lifetime of being careful with money can make them reluctant to run up the phone bill – even when it's yours.

Penny's mum Rene is 82. She lives a couple of hours away from the rest of the family.

'Mum will never chat. She phones us up once a week, says she and Dad are fine, asks how we are and then rings off. We've tried to get round it by making the calls ourselves, but just as you're settling down to a good gossip, she'll say goodbye! We've told her that we don't mind the money but she can't seem to help it!'

In this situation, try to call more often instead. Five minutes a couple of times a week can feel just as good as one half-hour call and will have the advantage of keeping you more immediately up to date.

As they get frailer, it can be a good idea to set them up with a mobile phone. Judy gave a phone to her 80-year-old mother Anne. She set up a pre-pay system and programmed the phone with important numbers like those of family members and the doctor's surgery.

'Dad didn't want anything to do with mobile phones, but he's got slight Alzheimer's so we knew it would have to be Mum. At first she was reluctant – said she wouldn't be able to cope. But we told her it was just in case anything happened to her or Dad, asked her if she wouldn't feel safer knowing she could always reach us, and said it would help put *our* minds at rest too. I'm sure she did it for Dad more than herself.

'I showed her how to use it and recharge it, and suggested she keep it in her handbag all the time so she'd have it with her and always know where it is. I ring her on it every now and then just to keep it in her mind.'

Alarms are another way of ensuring peace of mind for all of you. Local authorities usually run an emergency response system of some kind, or they'll provide you with the names of companies that do. An alarm unit is fitted to the phone, connected to a control centre that's staffed 24 hours a day. Your parents will probably have to pay for this – an installation fee and then a small weekly charge – but it can be very reassuring for them to know there's always someone at the end of the line. Help the Aged has a similar scheme called SeniorLink, and there are likely to be others in your parents' area too. Check costs though – they can vary.

Who's Doing the Caring?

If one of your parents becomes in need of help the other might end up taking on the whole burden. This is incredibly common – there are a staggering 1.5 million carers aged over 60 in the UK.

Being a carer isn't easy, especially when you're elderly yourself. There's help available to ease the burden but, as with so many of the local authority services, or grants and benefits, you have to know what to ask for – information isn't always volunteered. For example, literally hundreds of millions of pounds in benefits for carers go unclaimed every year. Elderly people can struggle on without the help they're entitled to, physical and financial, through not even knowing they are 'carers'.

This happened to Salma's parents, Anurag and Pinki, who were in their eighties. Pinki had several strokes, and over time began to need a lot of care.

'Dad looked after Mum – he just took it all on. They'd been married for sixty years so it seemed natural to him, but it was really too much. Mum needed a lot of attention night and day. She needed turning, she was incontinent, which meant a lot of laundry – the list went on and on.

'Dad wouldn't let us help except when we visited them, which we couldn't do very often anyway. He said Mum was his job. She didn't need to be in hospital so he just carried on. He got so tired that one lunchtime we found him asleep with his head on the kitchen table. Once or twice we got there in the morning to find Mum in a mess because she'd been incontinent in the night and Dad had been too tired to change her.

'We told their GP how worried we were, and he said that Dad and Mum could both have their own assessments, one for her needs, and one for his as carer. As a result he got some help with Mum's care, and they found they were both entitled to some financial help that no one had mentioned before.'

Local authorities must give carers their own separate assessment if they ask for one because they might be in need of help themselves, and at the very least their needs should be taken into account in any assessment of the person they're caring for. Contact social services if your parents are in this situation. How help will be administered varies across the UK, so check your parents' area. Various allowances are available under certain circumstances – it's complex, but they do exist.

If one of your parents is looking after the other, try to keep a close eye – it's an exhausting job being a carer and depression, anger, frustration and stress can all take their toll. Apart from the sheer hard work, there's the strain of being solely responsible for someone else's wellbeing and safety. It can be lonely and isolating.

They could be feeling trapped because they're afraid to leave the house in case something happens. And, however much they love their partner, there's likely to be a certain amount of resentment at all the demands made on them, and guilt because they feel they *shouldn't* resent it. They might also be feeling guilty because they're well and their partner isn't. On top of all this there's the general misery of seeing someone you love in such a helpless position.

Give them a chance to let off steam. If they can express their resentment and anger to you, safe in the knowledge that you understand and won't judge them, it will be an enormous relief.

See if you can give them a little change, like taking over so they can go out once in a while, even if it's only to the shops. Check that they're looking after their own health. Are they getting enough sleep, fresh air? Are they eating properly? If you think they're starting to lose ground you could talk to social services about another assessment.

If you or a member of your family is planning to take on some of the caring, be sure you think hard about what's involved beforehand. Stephanie's parents Hilda and Martin were both in their seventies when Hilda developed cancer. Stephanie became her part-time carer.

'At the weekends and on my days off from work I'd go up and stay over to give Dad a break and a night's sleep. I'd be looking after Mum all day and up with her half the night. The district nurse would come in the morning to wash her and get her out of bed, but I'd never know exactly what time she'd arrive and I'd have to wait for her, which would make me late for work. I couldn't have done it without Dad. He was marvellous, but even then it was a terrific strain.

'Mum was so dependent on us that she'd watch our every move. I couldn't leave the house without her asking where I was going – when would I be back? She was permanently afraid that she'd be left alone. I was so worn down, what with doing my full-time job and looking after Mum, that I'd go home to my husband and break down in tears.'

It takes enormous commitment to be a carer. Sometimes it can happen almost by default. One member of a family is in the right – or wrong – place at the crucial time and it just goes on from there.

Whether you're a close family or not, try to talk it through very carefully before it all gets dumped on one person – even if that person won't be you. It's a horrendous responsibility and can sour your relationship with your parent.

Janice's 73-year-old mother Janet had a series of severe heart attacks. When she came out of hospital, Janice, who was still living at home, became her carer.

'Before she was ill Mum had done the lighter housework because I was out at work all day. Now I had to do it all and care for her too. She needed help to go to the toilet, sometimes in the middle of the night, help getting in and out of the shower, her bed . . . she was heavy and I'm slight so it was extremely hard work. My whole life went on hold – friends, hobbies – even my boyfriend had to take a back seat. There was no time for anything except my job and Mum.

'Mum changed too. She went from a cheerful person to being bitter and cross all the time. And she was really selfish. If she wanted me to do something that she knew would be awkward for me, she'd act the martyr and I'd just give in.

'I loved her, but I started to hate her too. She took me completely for granted. My two brothers would just waltz in every couple of weeks or so with a bunch of flowers and a smile and you'd think they were heroes the way she went on. They could do no wrong, and it was galling because I was doing all the work.'

A good talk with her mother about how she felt could have worked wonders for both of them. Janet might have been making a fuss of her sons precisely *because* she didn't see them very often and wanted to make sure they kept on coming. Making a comparison probably never entered her head.

Janice lived with her mother so she wasn't expecting her brothers to take over, but if they'd sometimes taken Janet out for the day or each had her to stay with them for a weekend every few weeks it would have lightened Janice's load enormously. If she'd told her brothers how much work she was doing they might have agreed to take some of the strain. It's possible they didn't even realize what a carer has to cope with – few people do. But she'd have needed to tackle it calmly and without accusations, something that's not easy to do when you're at the end of your tether.

Instead, Janice's pent-up resentment came flooding out after her mother's funeral, and the family row that followed Janet's death turned it into a double tragedy. A chat with her mother might have opened up the way for Janet to get her fears off her chest. It could have put their relationship back on track.

If you're totally dependent on the goodwill of others you become very vulnerable. Am I too much trouble? Will they stop loving me? Do I matter enough to them or will they just walk away and leave me? Imagine it – you might well feel that emotional blackmail is the only way to keep people in your life. The irony is, of course, that behaviour of this kind can cause exactly what you're afraid of – it can drive people away.

You might have previously been totally secure in your relationship with your family or partner, but all that can change in these circumstances. You feel guilty because you're causing so much trouble and work, and angry with yourself for being in this state – maybe even resentful of your partner or family for not being ill, and ashamed of that resentment.

All this is quite enough to cause a major personality change, and it can be enormously important for families to realize this and make allowances, however mean your parents seem to have become. So often people say, 'He changed out of all recognition when he got old. He wasn't a nice person any more.'

Try not to let it change your feelings for them. Your memories of your parents will, eventually, be all you have left of them, and you want to remember them at their best, not their worst. If you can manage it, don't let them get to you.

Getting Things Organized

Charities like Crossroads exist to give carers a breather, and Help the Aged and Carers UK give advice and support. It's also not unusual for a family member or members to share the care with someone supplied by social services but, if this is the plan, make sure you all know what's supposed to be happening and when.

Neville's mother Gladys was 80 and lived just a few hundred yards away.

'She'd managed in her flat for years, then she developed cancer and became a lot more frail. We lived so near her I could go in every morning to make her some breakfast then pop up later in the day to see she was OK, and get her another meal. She didn't want me to help her with intimate things like dressing and bathing.

'I arrived at my mother's one morning to find a young girl who said she was there to "help" Mum. Neither of us had ever seen her before and we didn't know where she'd come from. She offered no explanation, just asked did I need her to stay, and when I said, "No, I can manage," she left.

'Sometimes when I went to Mum's this girl would be there and sometimes not. My mother never knew when, or if, she was coming and neither did I, so I'd get there and Mum might still be stuck in bed, or I'd arrive to find everything had been done.

'I didn't know what was supposed to be going on – I was new at this. When something happens to one of your parents you're thrown in at the deep end. It's a bit like having a first baby, there are no rules and you have no experience.'

'Then a bill arrived from a company that supplies personal care. My mother's doctor had talked to social services about her, they'd decided she needed extra help and contracted it out, all without telling her or any of us.

'I had no problem with social services arranging help. I just wish they'd talked to my mother – and me – about what they were doing. She was perfectly capable of understanding but nobody bothered to explain.'

'In any case Mum didn't like having a very young stranger coming and going at unpredictable times, and making it impossible for her to have a routine. It must have felt chaotic.'

It's worth checking what form your parents' personal care is going to take. If social services are contracting it out to a company, make sure your parents are happy with who they're sending in. You could find out, for example, if it will be the same person, or set of people, all the time. Your parents might find it unsettling never knowing who's going to turn up, or they could find the idea of meeting new people stimulating – it will depend partly on how frail they are.

Care workers, district nurses and other professionals can't always specify an exact time. Their timetable has to be flexible – but only up to a point. If you're helping with care you need to make it clear to your parent's care worker exactly when you can and can't be there, especially if you have a job. Otherwise you could find yourself hanging around for them to come and take over, or even having to decide whether to take a risk and leave your parent alone.

Local authorities are legally obliged to notify carers of their right to an assessment, even when the person they're caring for hasn't had one. What's more, they must take into account your own work commitments and hobbies.

Getting the right balance of care can sometimes be a bit of a marathon. Local authorities have a lot of help to offer, and generally speaking a huge amount of goodwill, but they're not always very good at communicating and might well not volunteer the things you and your parents need to know. The answer is to take the initiative and ask. The guides below give you an idea of what's usually available and where to go for specific information about your area, but they're just the tip of the iceberg.

Guide 1 – Who Pays for Care?

Every local authority has its own charging policy and it's very complicated, so always check. If you make assumptions you might be unpleasantly surprised. The best place to start is the Citizens' Advice Bureaux. SeniorLine 0808 8006565 and Northern Ireland 0808 8087575 also give advice. Local authorities shouldn't charge for NHS services.

Service	Who pays
Personal care: help with going to the toilet, dressing, overnight care, continence, bathing, laundry etc. What constitutes personal care could vary from one local authority to another	Means-tested in England and Wales – the cost shouldn't drop your income below a minimum level. Free in Scotland if you're over 65. Can be free in Wales but check local authority rules. Can be free in Northern Ireland if you're over 75 but check rules.
Cleaning and household tasks	In England and Wales you will probably have to pay if that's all that's needed. Means-tested if part of personal care package. Sometimes charged for in Scotland – check rules. Can be free in Northern Ireland if you're over 75 – check rules.
Meals	Means-tested.
Community care equipment: walking frames, toilet chairs, special beds, bathing equip-ment, wheelchairs	Should be free. If you want a specific wheelchair you may have to pay the difference.
Handrails, grab handles, small adaptations	Usually free up to a certain figure
NHS home services – district nurses etc.	Free

Guide 2 – Allowances, Benefits, Grants and Payments

This is a general guide to give you a start. Once again the CAB is a mine of information and should be the first stop. Millions of pounds in benefits go unclaimed every year, so persevere.

What benefit	Who gets it	Contact
Disability Living Allowance	Not means-tested. Depends on physical need. Can include a mobility allowance but this must be claimed before age 65	Benefits enquiry line 0800 882200 Northern Ireland: 0800 2206074
Attendance Allowance To help with cost of personal care	Not means-tested. Based on physical need	Benefits enquiry lines as above
Direct Payments Allows you to buy your own services direct	Means-tested. Discretionary. May be paid to carers too, but check it out – Scotland has different rules and other regions may vary	National Centre for Independent Living 020 7587 1663 www.ncil.org.uk N. Ireland: Centre for Independent Living East 02890 875001 West 02837 522282 Scottish Executive 0131 5585200

Continued overleaf

What benefit	Who gets it	Contact
Disabled Facilities Grants: loans, labour, materials, advice for adapting your home – bathrooms, stair lifts etc.	Means-tested. Discretionary. Don't start work until application has been approved	Home Improvement Agency England: Foundations 01457 891909 N. Ireland: Local disability advice project (see local phone book for number) Scotland: Care and Repair Forum: 0141 2219879 Wales: Care and Repair Cymru 02920 576286
Home Improvement Grants (Scotland)	Means-tested	Local council
Heating and insulation payments	Means-tested	England: 0800 3166011 N. Ireland: 0800 181667 Scotland: 0800 0720150 Wales: 0800 3162815
Winter Fuel Payments Help with heating costs	Not means-tested	Winter fuel payment helpline: 0845 9151515
Pension Credit Tops up pension	Means-tested	Great Britain: 0845 6060265 N. Ireland: 0808 1006165
Council Tax Benefit	Means-tested	Local Authority
Carer's Allowance	Means-tested	Carer's Allowance Unit: 01772 899729 N. Ireland: 02890 906186

Guide 3 – Home Alterations and Disability Equipment

There are a lot of charities and government run organizations to help with advice, leaflets etc. Here are some of them.

Organization	Help Provided
Disabled Living Foundation Helpline: 0870 6039177 www.dlf.org.uk Disability Action Northern Ireland: 02890 297880 www.disabilityaction.org Update Scotland: 0131 5585200 www.update.org.uk Disability Wales: 02920 887325 Helpline: 0800 7316282 www.disabilitywales.org Disabled Living Centres Council: 0161 8341044 www.dlcc.org.uk	Advice and centres to give you hands-on try-outs.
Ricability: 020 7427 2460 www.ricability.org.uk	Guides to equipment. Scooter measurement guides (will that scooter fit through your door?)
Remap: 0845 1300456 www.remap.org.uk **Demand:** 01923 681800 www.demand.org.uk	Charities that build specific equipment for individual needs
Disability Equipment Register: 01454 318818 www.disabilityequipment-register.org.uk	Buys and sells second-hand equipment. Produces a magazine
Home Improvement Agencies	See Guide 2
Centre For Accessible Environments: 020 7840 0125 www.cae.org.uk	Advice on alterations
Citizens' Advice Bureaux (see local phone book)	Advice on council grants

Guide 4 – Help for Carers

Organization	Help Provided
Carers UK Helpline: 0808 8087777 www.carersuk.org **Carers Scotland:** 0141 2219141 www.carerscotland.org **Carers Wales:** 0292 0811370 www.carerswales.org **Carers Northern Ireland:** 02890 439843	Advice for carers plus guides on every aspect of being a carer. Pressure group on behalf of carers.
Princess Royal Trust For Carers 020 7480 7788 www.carers.org	UK support network for carers.
Crossroads Association: 0845 1309177 www.crossroads.org.uk Northern Ireland: 02891 814455 www.crossroadscare.co.uk Scotland: 0141 2263793	Provides cover so carers can have a break
Carer's Allowance Unit: Great Britain: 01772 899729 Northern Ireland: 02890 906186	Benefit for carers (there are specific criteria).
Samaritans: 0845 7909090	24-hour helpline

Guide 5 – More Charities/Organisations

Organization	Help Provided
Talking Newspapers Association 01435 866102 www.tnauk.org.uk	Produces talking newspapers
Partially Sighted Society 01302 323132	Gives advice on equipment
University of The Third Age www.u3a.org.uk	Runs classes and organizes events on a variety of subjects
Independent Living Alternatives 020 8906 9265	Gives advice on hiring and employing your own helpers
Community Service Volunteers 020 7278 6601	Brings together volunteers and people who need help
Hospice Information Service 0870 9033903	Gives information on home nursing and respite care for the terminally ill
Help The Aged SeniorLine: 0808 8006565 N. Ireland: 0808 8087575	Provides booklets on various aspects of community care Helpline

Guide 6 – Making a Complaint

Complaint	Who to contact
Anything to do with your assessment – e.g. refusal to give one, long wait, don't agree with results. Anything to do with care provided – e.g. you don't think it's suitable.	Use the local authority complaints procedure. For advice on how to do this contact SeniorLine: 0808 8006565 Northern Ireland: 0808 8087575 To help you make a complaint contact CAB or Age Concern (see local phone book for both).
Concerning your NHS services	Ask for a copy of NHS complaints procedure. CAB will advise you. If not satisfied with the result complain to your local health service ombudsman – again, CAB will advise
If Attendance Allowance is refused or you feel the rate is incorrect	SeniorLine – as above CAB

At a Glance

- Keep in touch with your parents' GP and/or social services
- A carer is also entitled to have an assessment or their needs considered
- Ask what services are available
- Ask what financial help is available
- Discuss the caring setup with the whole family
- Give any family carers time off
- Encourage your parents to have new interests
- Be tolerant of any personality changes

Chapter 4

WHEN A MOVE IS INEVITABLE

It's been said you can judge a civilization by the way it treats the very young and the very old. If that's true it puts a few question marks in the margins of our own social history as far as the elderly are concerned. It's not so much that individuals or families don't care, it's more that the way society is structured makes it harder, rather than easier, for people to do anything practical about that caring.

The infrastructure of care for the elderly, and the way the state deals with the financial issues at both national and local levels, can make things even more difficult, sometimes in ways reminiscent of the Poor Law in the nineteenth century. If you can pay, you might get lucky – if you can't pay, you're effectively in the hands of your local authority, and your freedom of choice is at best severely limited. Move a hundred miles to be in sheltered housing nearer your family? Well, you'll have to go to the bottom of another waiting list. Don't like this care home? Sorry, there's nowhere else . . .

It's appalling that if you're a loser in the postcode lottery you can wait years (if you have years) for the right kind of local authority sheltered accommodation – or take what no one else wants.

It's terrifying that standards in residential care homes, both state run and private, can vary so widely.

It's shaming that elderly people have died while waiting for their finances to be correctly assessed by their strategic health authority – and that there's scope for faulty assessment.

It's worrying that scandals and scare stories concerning the care of the elderly appear so frequently in the media.

It's no wonder that we're inclined to stick our heads firmly in the sand when it comes to facing up to moving out of our own home. It can seem like hell waiting round the corner. Sometimes it takes a sudden cataclysmic event like a severe stroke or heart attack to bring us face to face with some hard decisions.

And there are plenty of other reasons for reluctance; it's a highly emotive area for everyone. Just the thought of breaking up your parents' home and depriving them of the final shreds of freedom can make you feel guilty. To your parents the thought can seem like surrendering their whole identity.

Then there's the question of what kind of care they'll need and where they'll live: With you or another family member? In sheltered housing? In a home? What kind of home? What will be best for them, and for you? What will they want, and what do you want? How much will it all cost and who'll pay?

This is the last step, and your parents know that every bit as well as you. From the decisions made now there's likely to be no going back. Your parents' happiness and your own peace of mind – now and long after they're dead – depend on tackling this as openly and carefully as possible.

It can be done. Local authorities aren't monsters, but they do have too big a workload and too few resources. They're stretched, often to the limit; they sometimes mess up badly, but mostly they do mean well, even when they're catastrophically bad at showing it.

Getting the Right Level of Care

If you begin to worry that your parents are losing their ability to cope at home, the best way to start is, as always, with your parents' GP, care worker or district nurse. Talk to your parents about your concerns and suggest an assessment. Once you alert social services or the NHS they should visit your parents anyway. They regard assessments as very much an ongoing process, and they'll give an expert evaluation of your parents' ability to continue caring for themselves at home.

They'll look at whether one or both of your parents need actual nursing, their physical and mental state (blindness, immobility or dementia, for example), and the suitability of the house they currently live in. If social services feel staying in their own home is no longer a possibility, the written assessment will specify the level of care they feel would be best.

Once your parents get their copy of this, suggest to them that you all sit down together with the social worker and talk about what's being put forward. Remind them they're not obliged to agree with the assessment. Explain that it will give them the chance to ask social services some questions, and say that you'll be asking questions too. A meeting like this is better than your parents being told things they might forget by someone you're never around to see. Tell them not to worry – nobody can do anything without their consent. Reassure them that they have the final say, and they can't be moved into sheltered housing, residential care – or in with you for that matter – against their will.

Have a lot of chats with your parents about what *they* want – and really listen to what they're saying. Encourage them to be honest, tell you frankly how they feel, not to

**worry that you'll be offended (try not to be). The truth is
what matters here.**

It's best if you can avoid giving your own views to start with,
then they won't feel you're pushing them in any particular
direction. You can say what you think later – or when they ask
you! What's important is that your parents feel unthreatened,
unhurried, and able to reach their own conclusion.

**Whatever the outcome and wherever they end up living,
it's vital to their peace of mind that they make the decision
themselves, even if they need help to do so.**

Of course, if their circumstances don't allow for much delay,
it's even more important for them to feel they've had the
opportunity to talk about it and come to terms with what's
happening.

It's worth bearing in mind that for families who don't get on
this can be a dangerous moment – a potentially permanent
fracture point. There are others ahead but this one's right up
there, so if you really don't want it to split the family atom,
keep talking to each other – your parents, your partner, your
siblings, their partners. Talk, talk and talk again, and listen a
lot. Shout at each other if you must, but get it out into the
open. It can make a truly amazing difference.

Sheltered Housing

This is a good setup if your parents are reasonably active but
nervous about living on their own any longer. Basically it's a
collection of small homes with a manager, designed for people
who can look after themselves as long as there's someone
around to keep an eye on them.

In sheltered accommodation your parents can keep their privacy but have the security of knowing there's backup if they need help. And they could be attracted by the possibility of a social life within the sheltered community – there is less chance of being lonely.

There are various levels, from the simple presence of a warden/manager to the kind that's known as 'very sheltered housing'. The choice would depend on how fit and independent your parents are. If they're already receiving a lot of personal care in their own home, for example, they might need the very sheltered kind.

Various organizations provide sheltered housing – private developers sell it, local authorities and voluntary organizations offer it for rent, and housing associations have homes to rent or part-buy. Whether they're renting or they buy outright, there will probably be a service charge to pay for repairs and running costs.

How your parents choose to go forward will depend on their financial situation. If they own their own home, unless they've got plenty of other capital they'll probably need to sell it to buy a sheltered unit, because although there can be exceptions, homeowners are very unlikely to be given a local authority place.

Polly's mother Enid was 84 when she sold her bungalow to buy a sheltered home near her daughter.

'Mum's thrilled to bits. The housing scheme is handy for the shops, and there's a tiny garden she enjoys looking after.'

Enid herself says she feels safe for the first time in a couple of years.

'I was getting very shaky on my legs – I've had a few funny turns and worried about being on my own. It's a relief knowing that someone's always there to keep an eye open and that

I won't have to drag Polly out of bed in the middle of the night if I have a fall or something.

'I love my little maisonette. It's smart and easy to look after, and I can still see my friends. I do my own cooking and have my bit of garden. I've still got a reason to get up in the mornings!'

The price Enid got for her bungalow meant she could go down this route. If your parents can't afford to buy, their choices are more limited.

Local authority sheltered accommodation can only be rented, and getting it isn't necessarily easy. Every area has its own policy about who gets what and many will have a minimum residency rule. This can make it difficult to move areas to be nearer to you or other family members. Even if they want to stay where they are, they might not end up with anything they like.

Waiting lists are very long in some places, especially for the best housing. You can sometimes rise up the list by agreeing, basically, to look at anything.

Presumably to ease their backlog and to help elderly people raise capital, some local authorities will buy back council houses that were purchased under the right-to-buy scheme, but be warned – they probably won't pay what the house would fetch on the open market, and your parents could still end up in rented council sheltered accommodation because their money won't stretch to anything else. It makes more sense for them to sell the house themselves for as much as they can and then decide how they want to spend the cash.

Whatever your parents' circumstances, it's best if they take financial advice before making any arrangements. They could either consult a solicitor or the Citizens' Advice Bureaux, who can advise on their rights and on local schemes.

In any case they'll need to look at the schemes available, private and otherwise, in the area they want to live. The standard will vary from fairly simple to luxurious, largely depending on cost. Make absolutely sure your parents know exactly what the various schemes cover, and what they'll be getting for their money.

If the value of your parents' home is insufficient to allow them to buy anything outright, then some housing associations will sell them part of a unit and they can pay rent on the rest.

Robert's 87-year-old father Steve wanted to move into sheltered housing when his wife died, but he didn't have enough capital.

'Dad said he didn't like the idea of us being forever worried about him, and he wanted to do things at his own pace and not be fussed over, so a sheltered scheme seemed the answer. We shopped around and finally found something he liked and could cope with. It's a housing association development and he's half-owner of his one-bedroom home. It's only a hundred yards from the town centre so he can walk to the shops and get anything he might need.

'Everything we looked at was so tiny, and that was a problem because Dad's furniture isn't small. Of course he knew he'd have to leave most of it behind, but even then it was a squeeze. It's upsetting.'

'He can't see well so his TV is big screen, and what with his walking frame and so on, by the time we got his sofa in the place was full. We could have bought him smaller furniture, but naturally he wanted to keep as many of his own things as he could. Almost everything had to go – it's such a comedown. He's accepted it because it's allowed him to continue to have a grown-up life, but it's upsetting for him too. It's the finality of it. He knows he won't be moving again.

'We're very bad at this kind of housing in the UK – there's very little decent accommodation for elderly people.'

Steve's experience is typical. It's ironic that so many of us spend a chunk of our working lives thinking that one day we'll sell up and buy a bungalow in a beautiful spot, then sit back to watch the world go by. It often doesn't work out like that because when we retire we decide that downsizing isn't an option – the house is getting full again, this time with visiting grandchildren, and it can seem like a bad idea to up sticks to the other end of the country to be among strangers just when we might start to need help.

As a result, for many elderly people a tiny flat or maisonette might be the first move they've made for many years, and it can come as a shock. Try to bear this in mind if your parents get emotional about what to take and what to leave behind. How would *you* choose? Help them stay calm about it by being calm yourself.

It can be a good idea to keep up your sleeve some of the things they don't take – pictures, ornaments, keepsakes – and produce them from time to time when the first trauma has worn off – 'I was going through a box the other day and look what I found'. Your parents will greet them with open arms.

Residential Care Homes

Moving into residential care can be some people's biggest fear – and it's not surprising. Quite apart from the difficulties of finding a good care home, the scare stories and bad public-ity, there are all the emotional and psychological factors.

As you get older your responsibilities seem gradually to melt away. Your children grow up, leave home, have families of their own; your grandchildren become too old to need babysitting; you retire from work. Relatives and friends of your own age start to die – the people who knew you when you were young and a force to be reckoned with are disap-pearing. Your world is shrinking.

The one place where you can still feel whole is your home. It's full of memories and, almost equally important, things – tangible reminders that you were once a person with a 'real' life.

'I can't go into a home – my things need me' – Maud, aged 80

Accepting the situation

If it becomes clear that residential care is the best way forward it's a good idea to sit down with your parents and talk it through. Whatever the professionals recommend, and what-ever you personally feel is the best option, try to approach the subject in an open-minded way. It's OK to stress the positive aspects – the freedom from anxiety, the comfort – but listen to how they feel about it. Give them space to voice their worries, and take their fears seriously. To you it may seem like the answer to all their problems, but to them it could feel like the end of the world.

Try to explore options, even if there don't seem to be many, and stay flexible. Your parents' dignity is one of the few things they have left, so at all costs avoid the phrase

'it's for your own good'. Remember how you felt as a child when someone said that to you.

Yasmin, who's 90, had a serious fall and had to move into a care home.

'I fell down the stairs and hurt myself badly. Neither of my sons could take me in so I ended up here. I understand – they can do without having to worry about me. And I don't mind really. I feel safe now and that's lovely.'

Yasmin has settled in well. She's come to terms with the move because she prefers having someone always there to care for her. Her family visits her often and her health actually improved because she stopped worrying.

Al's mother Caroline hasn't accepted it so easily. She came out of hospital straight into a care home with her husband Sylvester. She's 84 and several mini strokes have left her physically frail.

'Mum was in hospital for a few weeks, but as time went on it became increasingly clear that she wouldn't be able to cope at home and an assessment confirmed it. Dad was frail too, and she'd been looking after him.

'She kept on saying, "I can't look after your dad any more, can I?" She needed to hear us say over and over that she wouldn't be able to manage him.'

Caroline knew deep down that she had no choice, but constant reassurance was the only way to help her come to terms with it.

Sometimes your parents' reaction might surprise you. Lucy's mother Esther is 96. When she was 94 she announced that she'd decided to go into a care home.

'I was used to being on my own because I'd been a widow

for many years, but things were getting trickier and I wasn't cooking properly.

'I made up my mind suddenly – I thought, I've had enough, I'll go into a home. I just don't think it's fair to be a burden on your children. I've had my life and they're still living theirs.'

'I don't really like it though. I miss my garden, I'm stuck in my room a lot and I get bored – but I know I've got to be somewhere. You never expect it will come to you, but you might as well be practical. Life's cruel really; it seems endless. I think on the whole I'd have preferred to die when I was 90 – I was fine then. But I'm not miserable about it, what's the point?'

Esther has severe osteoporosis so she can't move about too easily. She can't see to read and this is a great sadness to her, but her extraordinary courage and pragmatism have helped her to accept what she sees as inevitable and it's clear that she's still able to get a kick out of life. She tends to see solutions rather than problems. There's no doubt that Esther's positive approach makes things easier for herself and her family.

Jim and Moira had a very different situation. Jim's mother Esme is 90 and her home was around twenty miles away from the rest of the family.

'Mum wanted to live with us. As she got less able to cope she kept on dropping hints about it. To be honest, we ducked out of confronting it for ages because we didn't fancy the idea, and even if we had it would have been impossible. We couldn't give her the constant care she needs.

'We felt guilty about it, as though we were neglecting her. It was awful because she kept on saying, "I won't be any trouble." We couldn't involve her in looking for a care home because she wouldn't entertain the idea at all. But we did a lot of research and finally found one we thought might suit her. We popped her into the car one day and took her to look at it. They were kind, gave us a cup of tea and introduced her to some residents. She started chatting and her face lit up.

'Taking mum to visit that home made all the difference. She saw she'd have company and something going on around her. We hadn't realized that one of the reasons she'd been so anxious to live with us was that she was lonely.'

Esme herself is the life and soul of her care home and she's philosophical about the changes to her life.

'Suddenly, I've got a set of new friends. I've gained hot food and company – but I've lost my village.'

She's a gregarious person and all her old friends have died so there was nobody to pick up the phone for a chat. When Jim and Moira showed her a home that suited her personality she relaxed quickly. Each home will have its own atmosphere and your parents need the best fit they can get if they're going to be really comfortable.

Who pays for a care home?

The first thing for your parents to do, before they even begin to look for a home, is to get a care assessment. This is vital if they want the local authority to pay – they won't get any funding without it. But it's important to have an assessment even if they're planning to pay for everything themselves, and then to choose a home that fits with it. This is because if their money eventually does run out and the local authority has to take over payment for their care home, they'll automatically assess them at that point, and there's no guarantee the assessment will result in your parents being able to stay in the same home – they could end up having to move.

Once they've been assessed, if your parents are intending to pay for their own care, they can get a list of homes that fit with the assessment, and go ahead and find one. If they can't afford to pay their own way they should tell the local authority, who will means-test their income and assets and decide how much, if anything, they'll have to contribute.

Below a minimum amount the local authority should pick up the tab; above a maximum figure your parents will pay for everything, and there's a sliding scale in between. It's very complicated, and each local authority has its own rules and interpretations. If both your parents are going into a care home they'll be financially assessed separately.

Try to keep an eye on the financial assessment. It's vital the sums are done correctly because your parents' home will be counted as an asset and, unless they have sufficient income to cover their care home fees, they'll be expected to sell it to use the money to pay for them.

There are exceptions to this. Under some circumstances the NHS will pay part – or even all – without a means test. It depends on whether your parents need nursing care, how much and what kind. However, the criteria are open to inter-pretation. There's a history of some strategic health authorities being too tough in applying the criteria and elderly people having to sell their homes unnecessarily to pay for care the NHS should have covered. Make sure your parents complain if there's any question at all of a mistake or they disagree with the decision.

Whoever is paying, the local authority shouldn't try to force your parents into a particular home. They have the right to choose – in theory – anywhere in the UK.

There are various rules, but broadly, provided the home they want fits their assessed needs, has room for them and doesn't cost more than the local authority's budget for that type of care, they should be able to go there. In practice this doesn't automatically happen.

Don't let the local authority put any pressure on your parents. In a world of waiting lists, complicated rules and busy people, they need your help to keep their end up and make sure they get their rights.

Where should the home be?

Location is an issue that needs to be resolved early on. For a start care home fees vary regionally, and if your parents want to move to an area that's more expensive they might not be covered for payment by the local authority unless their assessment states that a move is vital to their health and wellbeing.

If your parents already live near you they could stay in the area, keep contact with their friends and maintain as much of their old life as possible while still seeing you regularly. You'll all have the best of both worlds.

But if, as is so often the case, you all live a long way apart, things get more difficult. It's a fact that care homes aren't always what they should be, and if you're not nearby it will be difficult to keep an eye on the standard of care your parents are receiving.

From your parents' point of view it can effectively come down to a choice between keeping in touch with their friends or seeing a lot of their family. This is a hard one. Apart from the upheaval of the move itself, changing doctor, hairdresser, chiropodist, dentist, etc. will be exhausting and stressful for your parents, especially if they're frail. But if they stay where they are you're committing yourselves to travelling long distances to visit, which can be difficult to maintain.

Charlie's father Eugene is 78, and moved into a care home in the town where he'd lived for the last forty years.

'The home wasn't near any of us, but my sisters and I agreed between ourselves that we'd visit Dad roughly once a month each, which means he never goes more than a couple of weeks without seeing some of us. We don't have to feel guilty that we're not giving up every weekend to drive for hours to see him, and he keeps up with his friends. They can pop in any time, he gets taken out for the odd drink with them at his old club, and there's the constant stream of family visits, so everyone's happy.'

Eugene's family are all prepared to do their share but if you don't think yours will be so amenable, talk it over with them and try to come to some fair agreement. Your parents' continuing happiness will depend to a significant extent on feeling they're still a central and loved part of their family.

If everyone is spread out around the country your parents might well have strong views about whom they want to be near. This can be a real bone of contention. Whoever is going to be nearest might worry that the burden of visiting, and the attendant responsibility, is going to fall on them.

It's not unreasonable or selfish to be concerned about this. Uprooting them to be near you might sound fine – you'd be able to visit more often, they'd see their grandchildren, maybe come to stay with you sometimes. But with no nearby network of friends to fall back on, your parents' contact with people outside the home would effectively depend on you. You need to be honest with yourself – would you actually make those frequent visits?

Jessie is 87 and moved 300 miles to be in a care home near her elder son so she could see her granddaughters. Her younger son and her daughter haven't got children, and in any case they don't get on well with Jessie.

'A few months after I moved into the home my son and his wife split up. He took a job abroad and she moved back to where her own family live. It's 150 miles away and there's no way I can get there. I never see her or my grandchildren now – they've all forgotten me.'

Jessie's old friends can't travel to see her and she doesn't have the opportunity to make new ones outside the home, so she deeply regrets moving. Your parents will have their own opinion about where they want to settle and whether they want to move away from their home ground. Try to cover all the ramifications with them before they decide. It can help to make a list of pros and cons.

Finding the right home

There's no getting away from it, this is hard work for you and your parents, but good homes do exist. Once the area has been decided, the best way to start is to get a list of private and local authority-run homes that fit with your parents' assessed needs. There are also various websites and organizations that produce lists and advice, and government care standards authorities inspect every home in the country and publish reports. Talk to social workers and health visitors about the homes in the area and, most important of all, go and look at homes for yourself, and take your parents. Whatever you see in a brochure or on a website, nothing is as good as a visit.

Always turn up unannounced – there's a lot you can tell about a care home when nobody is expecting you. In fact, if a home insists on your making an appointment beforehand they may have something to hide.

Of course, if you ask them, care home managers are going to prefer you to make an appointment so they can ensure they'll be around to speak to you, but you can always arrange a proper meeting later. First impressions are what count. When you first step through the doors, start using your eyes, ears – and nose. What does it smell like? First thing in the morning, when residents are just getting up and their bedding and personal laundry is being dealt with, even the best home can smell a bit off – after all, some of the residents will be incontinent. But that shouldn't last all day. If the home is clean and the residents well cared for, by mid-morning any unpleasant odours should be long gone.

Look carefully at what's going on. Quite apart from whether the home is comfortably furnished and attractively decorated, what's the atmosphere like? Is it cheerful? Are there plenty of smiling faces? Do the residents look happy, engaged and stimulated or are they just sitting around staring into space?

Watch the staff – do the residents seem to like them? Are they warm and friendly or do they seem reserved? If you keep your eyes open there are dozens of small pointers to spot. Are they finding time to chat? Listen to the conversations – do you like the way they talk to residents? Do they address them with respect?

Do the staff speak English? This is important. Many homes employ staff from different countries, but they should be able to speak English clearly enough for residents to understand them. If you're elderly and deaf it can be difficult enough keeping up with what's going on around you without having a language barrier too. The reverse of this applies if English is not your parents' native language. They have the right to be in a home where their culture, religion and language are respected and taken into account.

Residents' rooms and general facilities will depend on the individual home but, again, they need to be clean, comfortable and odour free. Chat to the staff. Even if they're busy they should greet you pleasantly and make you welcome.

Later, when you get down to details with the manager, it's a good idea to check on the food. Is it tasty – does it look and smell tempting? Would you fancy it? Is there a choice? Are there good things for people on special diets? How regimented does everything seem? There are leaflets that suggest questions to ask (See Guide 4).

Don't be afraid to be tough and exacting when you're looking at prospective homes. Ask as many questions as you like. If the home objects to this, there's probably something wrong with it.

Try to take your parents to see as many places as possible, talk them through together immediately afterwards and take any reservations seriously. This is going to be their home for the rest of their lives, and they need to feel good about it.

If they're not well enough to travel around, or can't make up their minds, it can be possible for your parents to have a short stay in a home to see if they like it, although they'll have to pay for this.

Where a home is sited can make a terrific difference too. Your parents might like somewhere that's handy for the shops or the cinema. Is there transport? On the other hand they might prefer somewhere very quiet, with pleasant countryside or a garden where they can stroll in fine weather. They'll be happier somewhere that fits their emotional as well as physical and practical needs.

Making themselves at home

Any house move, whatever your age, is stressful, and this is a massive step for your parents, even if they're happy about it. Whether they're fairly well or pretty frail there are going to be aspects of their new life that will take some getting used to. You know how uncomfortable it can be when you first arrive at a holiday hotel – you feel disorientated, maybe a bit edgy, looking for things to criticize. And you're only going to be there for a couple of weeks. Imagine how it feels when you know you're moving into the place for good. People will try to reassure you, they'll keep telling you it's your home now – but basically you don't want it to be, so that's no comfort at all.

Your parents will have gone through an enormous amount of trauma to get to this point. They know there's no going back – they've probably had to sell their house and abandon most of their belongings. They're literally grieving for their furniture.

And they're grieving for their old life, their independence and responsibilities; they've lost so much. June was worried that her mother, 84-year-old Myra, couldn't settle in her care home.

'Mum was very listless. She wasn't eating and was clearly fretting. When I asked her what was wrong she said, "I want to go home. I don't like it here – I don't need my aprons." After a lifetime of working hard she couldn't get used to the idea that she had nothing to do.

'I had a word with the matron who arranged it so that Mum could give the staff a hand. She'd run a duster round, help set the tables for meals – light chores that were genuinely useful but within her physical scope. It made all the difference to her.'

As a society we tend to define ourselves by our role in life. Whether it's our career, or caring for our family, or both, who we are is what we do, and once that ceases we can feel useless, invisible, even nonexistent.

We all might fantasize about retiring to a life of leisure but, when it happens, many of us find the reality hard to come to terms with – and we've still got plenty of daily choices and chores. What if you can't choose?

What must it feel like to know that you *can't* ever again mow the lawn, do the washing up, peel a potato, make a sandwich, because you don't own a lawnmower, washing-up bowl, kitchen knife – a kitchen; that there's *nothing at all* you *have* to do, forever, until you die.

It sounds terrifying – and it is, because it means you're looking at the end of your life. Your parents may cope well and make jokes about it, or they may become depressed and say, 'I've come here to die.' If they're taking a while to settle in, you can do a lot to help them adjust by showing them you understand what they're going through.

Even caring families can brush aside their parents' unhappiness as inevitable, thinking there's no way to alter the basic fact – there they are and they'll need to get used to it. If they go on about it and moan every time you see them, try to be patient. Rather than being bracing and hoping they'll come to terms with it, be prepared to listen – over and over again if necessary. Let them talk it out, acknowledge their frustration, then reinforce the good aspects of their situation.

Moving into a care home involves learning a lot of new tricks at an age when this is hard to do. It's not simple to adapt to living with fifty other people if you've been alone or with just your partner. In fact it wouldn't be easy if you were young, would it? Coming to terms with communal living is a challenge for anyone and if you're old and infirm the tolerance, patience and understanding you need might be in short supply.

Visitors to the deaf old lady sitting in the chair next to you might have to bellow in her ear; the man with dementia might irritate you by shouting the same thing over and over again; squabbles might break out over favourite chairs or seats by the window. It's the school-playground syndrome, only this time there's no escape from it.

Things your parents wouldn't bother about in a normal busy life can assume different proportions in a hothouse atmosphere like this, and people who've always been easy-going and cheerful can become fussy, a bit obsessive and irritable. Your parents might not seem to be the same people – and you want them to be. Try to understand why they've changed.

The presence of residents with dementia, Alzheimer's and other mental problems can be deeply upsetting for those who aren't mentally frail.

'I don't want to stay here – it's full of old people' – Albert, aged 93

Albert isn't expressing a lack of compassion; he's simply making the distinction between himself and some of the people around him. It's important to him, as it is to all of us, to be his own person, an individual.

Getting some fun out of life

It's one thing to tell your parents they've earned a rest – so they have – but unlimited leisure is boring. If you can't see very well to read or watch TV, if you're rather deaf and find holding conversations a strain, then time is likely to hang heavily. Try to help them find ways of filling their days pleasantly.

'There isn't anything to get old for, really; it isn't worth the bother' – Nina, aged 90

If they're not too frail you could encourage them to take up new interests. A good care home will have people coming in all the time to talk to residents on all kinds of topics, maybe involve them in activities – crafts, painting, sing-alongs – things that give them something to think about and a reason to be in a certain place at a certain time. If that isn't happening you could talk to the manager and prompt a few ideas. You never know what you might set in motion.

Perhaps the home could ask a local historian or a school history class to come in and start a small project, something linked to the area or maybe to the Second World War years. There would be plenty of material from the residents – probably enough for a series of features in the local paper or on the radio. It would generate some excitement and turn back the clock to where your parents feel they really belong.

Immobility can be a big boredom factor. Molly is 85 and gets about indoors using a walking frame. She can't see well enough to go out on a motorized scooter, so she's stuck in the home for a lot of the time.

'I can't go out on my own and it's very frustrating because the town centre is only 200 yards away. I'd love to pop along and have a look in the shops or get a coffee, but there's nobody to take me. My friends come to see me but they can't do it – they're all as old as I am!

'The staff work very hard and have no time for themselves;

they can't spare the time to push me out in a wheelchair. It's a treat to see a good film or show, and my family try to take me when they visit.'

Molly's problem is a very common one. Being trapped indoors adds to the feeling of helplessness and hopelessness. If you live near enough to the home and your parents are up to it, you could collect them and bring them back to your house for the afternoon. This is a marvellous way of giving them a change of scene and keeping them involved in the family. Or perhaps take them out for lunch or on a short trip round the shops.

Instead of bringing them things they need like toiletries, new clothes and so on, try to take them to buy for themselves. Half an hour in Marks and Spencer could be the highlight of their week.

They'll enjoy it because it gives them back some choice. Yes, it's likely to tire them, but they'll have plenty of time to rest afterwards, and something to think about. If they're not up to shopping, try to walk them or wheel them round the garden for a few minutes.

If your parents had a hobby or interest when they were younger, you could try to keep it alive for them. Daisy is 83, and her care home is in the same town as her three sons and their families. She's been a widow for ten years.

'My husband used to take me dancing every week and my three sons and daughter know how much I miss it, so sometimes *they* take me! They waltz me round the floor a bit. I can't do much or stay very long but just being there with my toes tapping to the tunes is like being young again.'

Daisy looks forward to her dancing trips – they're an exciting contrast to the quiet life she leads, and give her a chance to put on her glad rags and have some fun. Her youngest son Nick is proud of her.

'It's wonderful to see how much she enjoys it. We love to see her eyes sparkle. She and Dad were great dancers in their day – they won competitions. We pull her leg and call her Ginger and she loves it.'

Daisy's children don't see why she should stagnate just because she's in a home. And everybody benefits – they all have a good time and it's keeping Daisy in their minds as she used to be, rather than what she's become. A couple of hours every few months are a small price to pay for the pleasure it gives her.

Enjoying a chat

Elderly people in a home can gradually sink into a kind of stupor if they're just left to sit about. You might notice, when you first arrive to visit your parents, that they can seem lethargic, not very alert, but that as you talk to them they brighten up and start to chat.

That's a sign they need stimulation. However housebound they were in their own home, their day would have involved people from outside. They'll be missing the contact they had with the milkman, the postman, the girl delivering the telephone directory.

'Thank you for talking to me – it's made me feel like a real person' – Aggie, aged 87

It's noticeable how people in care homes will perk up if even a stranger sits down for a quick word with them. They're desperately looking for something to vary their day, someone with a new perspective.

Virginia is 85 and her care home has a high proportion of residents with mental problems.

'There aren't many people I can have a conversation with – they don't remember what's just been said. I know they can't help it but it leaves me very isolated. I'm delighted when someone else's visitor comes to have a word.'

The staff at Virginia's home are wonderful. They haven't fallen into the habit that many care homes have of talking to all the residents as though they're not quite all there. It comes from compassion, not contempt, but even so it can be very demoralizing.

When you go to see your parents, remember they depend on you for news and topics of interest. If you've ever spent time in hospital you'll know how, once you've gone through your latest symptoms and treatment, you've really got nothing much new to say – you're depending on your visitor to give you all the gossip. Think how you'd run dry if you were in there for years. Not very much will have happened in your parents' daily lives worth talking about, so it's up to you to make the running. There are ways of giving them something to ask and talk about.

Joyce's grandfather Martin is 81 and has been in a care home for two years.

'From the start we've tried to keep things happening. In between visits we phone a lot – just quick, casual chats to keep him up to date, so he knows he's still involved. We send him pictures all the time – digital printouts of us doing ordinary everyday things and his great-grandchildren mucking about in the garden. They make cards for him and write him wobbly letters. The post is something for him to look forward to.'

It's important too, because it means the visits are pleasanter for Joyce and the family. Making one-sided conversation is hard work, and that in itself can put families off visiting very often.

Over time your enthusiasm for visiting might wane, but try not to go less often – it's desperately important for your parents. Iris is 89 and has been in her care home for three years, and she's very aware of this danger.

'My children and grandchildren all live too far away to visit me very often, but I know they visit when they can so I don't twist their arms to come and see me. If I acted disappointed or hurt I might put them off, so when they visit me I'm always cheerful and show them how pleased I am to see them.'

'I think they're grateful for that. My grandsons are lovely. We have a laugh and they really talk to me, about life, sport, politics – anything. My own mother used to get cross when we visited her. She'd cry and ask why we hadn't been sooner. I know from experience that it puts you off and you don't go as often or stay as long.'

Iris has been through it herself and she's determined not to fall into the same trap. In fact she's a happy person who makes the most of life and her family love her to bits. But she's quite right.

What must it be like to be so vulnerable – to be afraid that if you're not on your best behaviour those you love might abandon you?

Couples and care homes

If both your parents are alive the care home question can get complicated. Some only take people who need personal care, others provide nursing, but not all of the latter will cater for every kind of patient. This variation can pose a problem if your parents have been assessed as needing different kinds of care. The home they choose will need to be capable of looking after them both – and be willing to do so. If your parents are paying for everything themselves they need to make sure the homes they consider will deliver what's needed, and can continue to deliver if their health deteriorates.

If the local authority is paying, social services will try to find a home that will take your parents as a couple despite their differing needs. But if there are no places, or local homes can't deliver then they could end up being separated – maybe even a fair distance apart, because if all else fails social services will have to give priority to their individual needs and place them in homes accordingly.

Budget considerations can be a factor too. If a home that's appropriate for both your parents costs more than the local authority normally pays then they're not necessarily going to agree to cover the higher figure. They can suggest the family tops up the cost, although they can't force you to do this.

Local authorities try to be flexible and hopefully it doesn't happen too often, but cases of separation do occur. As so often, financial constraints and waiting lists vary from area to area.

This kind of forced separation can be a catastrophe for your parents – they could literally pine away. If you've lived with your partner for half a century or more it can feel as bad, if not worse, than their dying. To be effectively trapped, with no means of getting to your partner, yet knowing they're just a few miles down the road, is an appalling deprivation.

Visiting each other can be extremely difficult unless family and friends can provide transport. A short meeting, even once a week, isn't going to make them happy after a lifetime of living together. If your parents want to stay together and they find themselves sent to different homes, or it starts to look likely that they will be, take up the cudgels and complain.

It's possible too that one parent might be assessed as needing residential care and the other not. Again, if your parents are paying and they want to be together, they can choose a home that will take them both. But local authority-funded places can be in short supply, so one parent might be left behind to be cared for at home.

Under these circumstances social services might suggest very sheltered accommodation as a way of keeping your parents together. Whatever's put forward, try not to let them be pressured into anything they're not happy with.

It's possible of course that if one of your parents has been caring for the other they might be relieved to have the responsibility lifted from their shoulders. But even if that's the case the home still needs to be near enough for them to visit easily and as often as they want. This is crucial to the ongoing health and happiness of your parents – a strong argument when it comes to dealing with social services.

Coping as a couple

There are benefits from being in a home together. The roots of their existence – each other – are still intact so they won't feel so lonely. They can share worries and memories, talk things over and reassure each other just as they've always done. But that doesn't necessarily mean everything in the garden will be rosy. Women tend to live longer than men, and as a result care homes have a preponderance of women residents and far fewer married couples.

This can mean couples can be rather isolated – the other

residents mightn't like to disturb their privacy or interrupt, so they could end up sitting alone together and missing out on the social aspects of living in a community. A good home should help them to integrate.

You can do a lot when you visit by drawing other residents into your conversation and having a general chat – in other words treating it like a house party rather than behaving as if you were in a hospital dayroom.

There can be other problems too. Up until now their lives have revolved around caring for each other. Whether or not your mother had a job, her life will probably have been spent caring for your father. Giving up her role can take some getting used to.

Beryl's mother Lillian is 85. She and her husband Ira moved into a home together after he had a series of mini strokes.

'Mum had been looking after Dad at home for several years and when they moved into the care home she just carried on. She wouldn't let the staff do their job and tried to do it all herself. Dad would fall out of bed in the middle of the night and she'd struggle to lift him back. She's tiny and it was impossible for her, but she wouldn't push the emergency button. She said she didn't want to be a nuisance and anyway Dad was *her* responsibility.

'The staff told us about it and asked us to explain to her that they were there to look after Dad – it was what they were paid to do. The lack of sleep and the worry was affecting her health. We talked to her but it made no difference, she couldn't let go. Then Dad got ill and they moved him into a room next door to Mum so she could get some sleep. At first she was always getting up in the night to go in and see to him, but gradually she got more used to it and things improved. It wasn't until Dad died, though, that she really began to settle down.'

Lifelong habits are hard to break, and Lillian felt displaced, even resentful, that someone else was doing things for *her* husband. It's not necessarily logical but it's completely understandable. How would you like it if strangers suddenly started to invade your marriage and take over what you saw as your role? It's another example of the loss of control that comes with old age. In Lillian's case the home understood what she was going through and did a deal with her – she could do certain things for Ira if they could do others.

While a couple can be a great consolation to each other, they can also hold each other back. Phil's parents, Connie and Ernest, were in their eighties when they moved into a home together.

'They had a nice double room and it was a very pleasant home, but they moped. Dad was blind and couldn't walk, and Mum wouldn't go anywhere without him so she was effectively housebound too.'

'Mum never got any fresh air. The staff would offer to take her round the garden but she wouldn't often leave Dad, not even for a minute or two.

'We'd occasionally persuade her to come outside with us for five minutes but she'd never settle. We'd have liked to take her shopping or out for lunch. Dad would have been quite happy for her to go but she'd always say, "Who'll stay with your father?"'

Connie didn't want to acknowledge that Ernest would be OK without her, because it would have meant that she wasn't needed. She was effectively ignoring the fact that they were in a care home, trying to live as though they were still in their own home together. They'd had a long retirement and had gone for a walk most days so she found it hard, too, to enjoy a simple stroll without him.

Phil got round this by giving his mother specific reasons for going out with him: to shop for his father, perhaps. He found that if he set a time limit – back in an hour, for example – she'd brief Ernest on what was going to happen, give the staff a lot of instructions, and leave him more happily. She'd still fret, but it gave her a break.

Moving in with Family

This can be a happily-ever-after solution or a genuine nightmare, and it's another potential time when families fall out for good. For a start, whom do your parents want to move in with – and does that person want to take them? Whoever they live with is going to find it makes a tremendous difference to their lives, in big ways and small, and they're going to need to be prepared for this.

Warren says he'll have his parents and/or parents-in-law to live with him if they become unable to look after themselves.

'They haven't reached the age where it's an issue yet, but I'd do it for all four of them if it came to it. You can't put them in a home can you – they'd die there.'

This is a wonderful sentiment, but it needs a lot of thinking through.

However much you and your parents love each other, you're *all* going to need a phenomenal amount of tolerance and give and take if living together is going to work.

It might seem relatively simple for them just to move into your spare bedroom, but privacy could quickly become an issue for all of you.

98

Vishnu was 84 when he moved in with his son Chandra and his family.

'It seemed like such a good idea. We had a spare room and got on well with Dad, but it was much harder than we thought it would be. He was always *there*, sitting in the living room. We had to conduct our lives around him. We never had any privacy and couldn't even have a conversation on our own unless we escaped to the kitchen or the back garden. His bedroom was next door to ours so we had to whisper when we were in there. We wanted him to be happy, but our lives seemed to change completely – and for the worse.

'He had a TV in his bedroom but he wanted to be with us all the time. He'd sit watching his favourite programmes with the sound up loud. Nobody else could choose a channel, especially the kids. It drove them mad because he'd moan about the noise from their music and the way they clomped around the house. They're teenagers – they're not going to be quiet all the time.

'He'd been living with us for nine months when he had a stroke and went into hospital, where he died within a couple of weeks. We were terribly sad of course, but I honestly think if he'd still been living with us we'd all have ended up hating each other.'

Chandra knows his father didn't mean to be selfish, but when you've been used to living on your own it can be hard to adapt to someone else's life and habits. It was natural too that he didn't want to spend all his time upstairs in his bedroom, but there was nowhere else for him to go. He was probably feeling a bit strange and uncomfortable about being a 'guest', so if Chandra had started by asking him how *he* felt, it might have opened up the way for the air to be cleared for everyone.

And if they'd talked before he moved in about what it

would be like, everyone would have had an idea of what to expect. Vishnu probably didn't realize just how noisy living with teenagers can be, and if Chandra had told him he'd have had time to decide whether he really wanted to live in that environment or not.

Laying down some ground rules right at the start would have helped. Chandra could have pointed out that space was limited, and asked his father if he minded letting them have the living room to themselves two or three evenings a week. There would have been things that Vishnu would have liked to ask for too – perhaps for his grandchildren not to play music at certain times.

It's important for your parents to feel it's their *home*, and they're not there on sufferance. After all, it cuts both ways – they need their privacy too.

If you've got children living at home it's only fair to talk the idea through with them before you broach the subject with your parents – it will affect them profoundly. Ask them how they feel about it and explain that they're going to need to be understanding and tolerant – and do their bit to help you.

Before any decision is made, discuss all the ramifications with your parents. It's worth coming to an agreement about the arrangements because it could save arguments later. Will they have their own key? What about the kitchen – will they be able to make meals or snacks for themselves or are they eating with you? Two women in one kitchen can be a disaster unless it's planned for. Just imagine your mother, accustomed all her life to cooking for her family, having to come to terms with the fact that she's not the one in charge . . .

Of course it might not be safe for them to cook for themselves anyway, but whatever the circumstances, you need to get all this out in the open before you start. Talk in detail – it will throw up things none of you had thought of. Have a laugh about it if you can, but it's best not to duck the issues if you really want it to work.

And how does your partner feel about it? In fact, who's going to be doing all the work? With the best will in the world, having elderly parents living in your home is going to mean more work for *someone*, and you need to discuss who that someone is going to be. If one of you is at home all day then it's going to be them. On the other hand, if both of you are out at work, will your parents need outside help?

Having your parents to live with you is a big responsibility and unless other members of the family are prepared to do their share rows are very likely to develop. Before any of you agrees to take it on, try to get a commitment that the others will take some of the strain.

Win is 86 and has three daughters spread around the country. She's based with her eldest daughter Vicky, but spends two or three months with each of her other daughters every year to give Vicky a couple of long breaks.

'We've got the biggest house so Mum lives with us the most. She has her own bedroom and bathroom and we turned the study into a little sitting room for her. It's not so easy for my sisters – they've only got a bedroom free for her and sometimes I have to twist their arms a bit, but they do have her to stay.

'Mum spends a lot of her time in her own sitting room, but joins us for all her meals. She's no trouble really but she tries to be a help, which can be wearing. I'm glad to have a break sometimes to be honest.'

This is a good arrangement for everyone. Win has the

security of a permanent home plus the variety of a 'holiday' a couple of times a year, and nobody feels they're having to do it all.

Although Win is too frail to live alone she can manage to do a lot of things for herself. If she needs more help she'll be able to have a care worker, but some of the responsibility will inevitably fall on Vicky, who works full time.

This is something else that families – and parents themselves – need to take into consideration before any decision is made. Your parents may be fine now but circumstances change. Their physical and/or mental health could deteriorate. What would you do if that happens? Would they be prepared to go into a home? Would they expect to remain with you? Could you cope with this? The plain truth is that whatever outside help you might get, the very fact that your parents are in your home can become a big worry if you're not there constantly to keep an eye on them.

Judith's father Theo lived with them in their bungalow for six years.

'We gave up the dining room for him to have as a bedroom and he fitted in with us really well. Of course it wasn't perfect but my view has always been it's our job to look after our parents, not shove them into some home and forget about them. I wouldn't want my children to do that to me. It's a good job I felt like that because my brother wouldn't have had Dad. He said I was mad to take it on.

'We had six really good years. The kids loved him and he'd spend hours with them – he had so much patience. Then when he was 80 he had a bad stroke that left him partially paralysed. When he came out of hospital he needed a care worker both night and day, and that's when it became a strain.

'The carers were lovely but very young, and Dad hated the idea of "chits of girls" doing intimate things for him. He'd get cross and send them away. I could understand how he felt, so I ended up doing a lot of it.

'After six months I was worn to a frazzle and I finally talked to Dad about going into a home. He didn't really want to go but he knew his health was getting worse, so he agreed. He's such a lovely man. He said he didn't want the kids to have to cope if an emergency happened.'

'I still feel guilty that we ended up putting him in a home, but I don't see what else I could have done. He really needed 24-hour care and we couldn't give him that.'

It's natural for Judith to regret what happened, but she needs to remember that she gave her father six happy years with his family, and be glad about that. Her father doesn't resent it and she knows he understands.

Adapting your home

Depending on your parents' health and mobility you may need to make alterations to your home before they can come to live with you – something else to take into consideration at an early stage. Changes could be as simple as stair rails, or more complicated and expensive, like a stair lift or even an extension.

There are grants available under some circumstances, but as always there will be a means test. Your parents might contribute to the alterations if they can afford it, but this can be yet another contentious area if the rest of the family sees you as benefiting in ways they won't.

The alterations may add value to your home but, depending on what and where they are, they might actually detract from it. Stay as calm as you can. It will be difficult enough for your parents to talk about what's going to happen to their cash after they die, without having to watch their children scrapping about it while they're still alive.

Morris and Nora extended their house to accommodate Nora's mother, Marina.

Nora says:

'Mum had a couple of mini strokes and was getting frailer. She also became very deaf and we started to worry about her living alone. She wouldn't have been able to hear a smoke alarm.

'We had to move anyway because Morris changed jobs, so we looked for something we could extend. We built a ground-floor granny flat with a lounge, bathroom, kitchen, bedroom – even a little dining room, and its own front door. She was independent but we could keep an eye on her.

'Mum and Morris got on well and we saw a lot of her but were careful not to get into routines. We didn't always invite her for Sunday lunch, for example – we'd vary it. Otherwise she might have got too dependent and started to expect it and we wanted to be freer than that.'

Marina lived very happily for years in this way, only needing a care worker for a few months before she died. Building the annexe made life more pleasant and safer for Marina – and it simplified things for Morris and Nora too, and relieved them of worry. The flat is self-contained so hasn't had an adverse effect on the layout of the house as a whole, something that can happen if extensions or alterations aren't thought through carefully.

If you do decide on a granny-flat arrangement, it's worthwhile discussing the financial aspects of living together before you start. Are you going to divide the utility bills? How?

When Davina's 80-year-old mother Gwen became frail, she and her husband Errol converted their study into a bedroom and bathroom for her, and extended into the garage to give her a little sitting room.

'She was very proud and independent so we had gas and electricity meters installed. We didn't want her sitting in the cold, afraid to put the heat on in case it cost us too much. Errol used to go and read the meter and then give her a "bill" based on the reading. She was delighted to pay it – she didn't want to be beholden to us in any way. She had her own phone line too.'

Davina and Errol's thoughtfulness paid off for Gwen. It enabled her to keep her self-respect and feel she wasn't being a burden by paying her share.

Buying together

Going into any kind of joint financial arrangement needs careful thought, but it's especially true if you're planning joint home ownership. Ray's mother Sophie was 79 and had been a widow for a couple of years.

'Mum lived a long way from all of us and we wanted her to move, so we had a family powwow. My sister wanted to move to a bigger house and she suggested to Mum that she help to buy it and then move in.

'We all agreed it was a good idea but then we found that the house my sister fancied was in the middle of nowhere. Mum would have been stuck down a lane. She couldn't drive and there were no shops within walking distance. The rest of us put our foot down and we all fell out a bit with my sister, who hadn't really been thinking about Mum at all, just herself.'

This kind of arrangement can work, but your parents will need to think hard about their will, or things could get complicated later. Denise's father Eric was 79 when he bought a house with her.

'Dad sold his bungalow and came to live with us while we looked for a good house to buy together. My brothers went mad. They didn't see why I should get my share of Dad's cash straight away and wanted him to give them some money too, but he refused. He hasn't spoken to them for three years and he's threatening to cut them out of his will altogether. If he does that my brothers will never speak to me again – I'm in the middle of it and it's horrible.'

Jealousy can flare up fast and the results can be long lasting. Eric regarded his financial plans as *his* business, and didn't see why he should make any explanations, but if he'd sat down with his sons and told them what he was planning to do, they might have been more relaxed about the future. It would have made things easier for Denise too.

Buying together can work as long as you get on well, but there's always a chance your circumstances will change.

Dawn and her husband Bill bought a house with Dawn's 78-year-old mother, Beth.

'Mum was already staying with us but our house was too small and it didn't really work. We're good friends – Mum's been divorced for years and we've always relied on each other – but there just wasn't enough space and we got on top of each other. We all knew it wasn't a long-term solution. She and Bill got on, so we decided we'd be able to buy a nicer house if all three of us pooled our cash. I don't think we'd have even considered it if we'd had children; as it was it seemed the perfect answer.

'We found a house that could give us self-contained accommodation. Mum has her own bedroom, bathroom, kitchen, living room and, most important, her own front

door. It means she can come and go as she pleases and be completely independent.'

'We blocked the internal access between the two parts of the house and we've always respected each other's space. Mum doesn't just wander in – she waits to be asked, and I do the same with her, although we do see each other almost every day.

'I was looking for a cleaner and Mum volunteered to do it. I said OK, but only if she let me pay her the going rate. The result is that I've got a fantastic cleaner and Mum has a part-time job.'

Things were going well until Dawn's marriage started to fall apart. Beth began to feel uncomfortable.

'I was concerned about my daughter's happiness but, at the same time, I couldn't help wondering what was going to happen to *me*. What if they sold the house? It would have been very awkward financially. I didn't want to be selfish, but I had nowhere else to live and it worried me.'

Dawn admits that seeing how her mother was affected added to the stress she was going through with her marriage.

'When we divorced I bought Bill out and now there's just Mum and me. We're mates – we go out for days and on holiday together sometimes, but we never take anything for granted. We know when not to encroach on each other's life.'

Dawn and Beth have a good relationship based on mutual respect. Living together has made them closer than they were before. They're lucky – but they're prepared to work at it.

Whatever form of move your parents are thinking of making, they'll need your help to do the research. The guides below are a good starting point, and the main thing is to persevere. Elderly people often don't have the stamina for prolonged investigation, or for chasing elusive professionals.

Guide 1 – Sheltered Accommodation: What's Available?

Provider	Type
Local Authority	Solely for rent. Means-tested. Allocation policies and waiting lists vary regionally. Homeowners not given priority
Housing Associations	For rent/part-buy. Means-tested. Homeowners not given priority. Some offer the chance to part-buy and pay rent on the rest if you have insufficient capital to buy outright
Voluntary Organisations	Solely for rent. Have their own allocation policies
Private Developments	To buy

Guide 2 – Advice on Sheltered Accommodation

Type of Accommodation	Organisation	What it does
Local Authority	HOMES Mobility Scheme 020 7963 0200 www.homes.org.uk	Helps if you need to move areas to be nearer family.
Housing Association	Elderly Accommodation Counsel: 020 7820 1343 www.housingcare.org	Charity offering advice and lists of housing association schemes anywhere in UK, including very sheltered housing
	Citizens' Advice Bureaux Local phone number	Gives advice on schemes and finances
Voluntary Organizations	Abbeyfield Society 01727 857536 www.abbbeyfield.com	Charity with rented homes, plus meals
	The Almshouse Association 01344 452922 www.almshouses.org.uk	For a list of charities running alms-houses locally
	Elderly Accommodation Counsel as above	Lists of voluntary schemes
Private Housing	Retirement Homesearch England/Wales: 0845 8805560 Scotland: 0141 2482846 www.retirementhome-search.co.uk	Free service matching people looking for sheltered housing with what's available
	Elderly Accommodation Counsel as above	Lists of private schemes
Private Housing (new)	National House Building Council 01494 735369 www.nhbc.co.uk	If the builder is registered you'll be covered by NHBC sheltered housing code

Guide 3 – Care Homes: Where to Look

There are a lot of websites listing care homes, some sponsored.

Organization	What it Does
Local Authority	Provides a list of all homes – private and state run – in the area
Age Concern (see local phone book) www.ageconcern.org.uk	Provides list of local care homes
Care Standards Authorities www.csci.org.uk	Provides list of care homes in the UK
Counsel And Care 0845 3007585 www.counselandcare.org.uk	Gives advice on how to find a care home
Elderly Accommodation Counsel 020 7820 1343 www.housingcare.org	Provides list of care homes in UK

Guide 4 – Finding a Good Care Home

Organization	What They Do
Care Standards Authorities: England – Commission For Social Care Inspection: 0845 0150120 www.csci.org.uk N. Ireland – Dept of Health and Social Security: 02890 522028 Scottish Commission For The Regulation Of Care: 0845 6030890 www.carecommission.com Care Standards Inspectorate For Wales: 01443 848450 www.csiw.wales.gov.uk	CSAs inspect all care homes in the UK and issue twice-yearly reports on how they conform to national minimum standards. You can ask for a copy of the report on any home you're interested in.
Counsel And Care 0845 3007585 www.counselandcare.org.uk	Provides fact sheets, advice and guides.
Help The Aged SeniorLine: 0808 8006565 Northern Ireland: 0808 8087575	Provides housing advice and information. Ring SeniorLine for list of booklets.
Age Concern Local phone number, also England: 0800 009966 www.ageconcern.org.uk N. Ireland: 02890 325055 www.ageconcernni.org Scotland: 0845 1259732 www.ageconcern-scotland.org.uk Wales: 02920 431555 www.accymru.org.uk	Provides information, fact sheets.

Guide 5 – Care Homes: Who Pays?

Who's Paying?	How it works
Local Authority SeniorLine 0808 8006565 (Northern Ireland 0808 8087575) Help the Aged Care Fees Advice Service 0500767476 Age Concern have leaflets England: 0800 009966 www.ageconcern.org.uk Northern Ireland: 0289 0245729 www.ageconcermi.org Scotland: 0131 2203345 www.ageconcernscotland.org.uk Wales: 02920 371566 www.accymru.org.uk CAB local phone number	Funding policies vary locally – ask for a copy of the rules. You must have a care assessment first. They'll look at your income and capital and include the value of your home (except in certain circumstances – ask your local authority). Below a minimum figure the local authority pays for everything – they'll tell you what they'll pay and give you a list of homes that fit your needs and their price range. Above a maximum figure you pay for everything – they'll give you a list of homes that fit your needs. In between there's a sliding scale.
You Help The Aged Care Fees Advice 0500 767474 (free calls) Advice on managing your money to pay for your care home	You pay if you have above a maximum amount of assets, including the value of your home.

Who's Paying?	How it works
NHS Contact your local authority. SeniorLine has advice and leaflets.	Non-means-tested help with your care if your assessment says you need nursing care. But policy on who qualifies varies throughout the UK. Fully funded NHS care also exists, called continuing NHS care. Ask for an assessment. Very complex criteria.
Third party top up Contact your local authority.	The local authority won't fund you if you choose a home that is more expensive than their maximum for the level of care you've been assessed as needing, if there are spaces available in a cheaper suitable home. A relative or charity can make up the shortfall for the home of your choice. The local authority can't insist on a third party paying, but if you go down this route make sure the contributor can continue to pay – if they stop contributing the local authority may move you somewhere cheaper. If there are no suitable cheaper places available then the local authority should increase their payment.

Guide 6 – Couples and Financial Assessments

Age Concern and Help the Aged have various leaflets (see guide 5), and the CAB will give advice – they'll be in your local phonebook. Policy could vary regionally

Situation	What Happens
If you're both going into a home	You'll be assessed separately. Joint savings with your spouse will be classed as a set percentage each, regardless of what they actually are.
If one spouse is going into a home	Only that person is assessed. The local authority has no right to assess the other partner – BUT they can ask the spouse for a contribution and if he/she refuses they can take him/her to court for it. Policy on this varies locally. If only one spouse is going into a home the other won't have to sell the house if he/she is still living in it. Check local authority rules.

Guide 7 – Choosing a Care Home: Your Rights

Query	Solution
Can you choose a home if the local authority is paying?	Yes, provided your choice has a place for you, fits with their assessment of your needs, costs no more than the local authority's budget and will agree to the local authority's conditions.
If the local authority is paying can you move outside your area?	Yes, the above applies.
If the local authority is paying and your partner is going into a home and you are not?	Yes, the above applies but the home should also be near enough for you to visit easily. If you cannot afford to visit you may be entitled to travel expenses.

Guide 8 – Moving In With You: Grants and Benefits

Take a look at the guides at the end of chapter 2 for more advice.

What's On Offer	How It Works
Small alterations – grab rails etc. Talk to local authority	Free up to a maximum amount
Disabled Facilities Grant – help with building extensions, bathroom, shower room etc. Disability Rights Handbook 02072478776 www.disabilityalliance.org	Means-tested (the elderly person, not the family they will be moving in with). There will be an assessment by the local authority occupational therapist first. Policies on who qualifies vary
Council Tax	If a single person's parents move in with him/her, then that person's council tax could go UP. Check with the local authority
Winter Fuel Payment	Not means-tested. If there's anyone in your home over 60 then this payment goes directly to them – but only one payment per household
Benefit Enquiry Line 0800882200 Northern Ireland 0800220674	Queries on disability entitlements

Guide 9 – Financial Advice

Organization	Solution
Financial Services Authority 0845 6061234 www.fas.gov.uk	Government watchdog Fact sheets available
Charity Search 0117 9824060	Gives advice on charity funds

Guide 10 – Complaints/Your Rights

Organization	What it Does
Age Concern Advice Information And Mediation Service 0845 6002001	Complaints or queries about your rights, plus mediation
Local Government Ombudsmen England: 0845 6021983 www.lgo.org.uk Northern Ireland Ombudsman 0800 343424 www.ni-ombudsman.org.uk Scottish Public Services Ombudsman: 0870 0115378 www.scottishombudsman.org. uk Public Service Ombudsman for Wales: 0165 6641150 www.ombudsman-wales.org	These are independent arbitrators
Citizens' Advice Bureaux (see local phone book)	Provides information on how to complain
Relatives and Residents Association Advice line 02073598136 www.relres.org.uk	Information and advice on your rights
Action on Elder Abuse Helpline UK: 0808 8088141 www.elderabuse.org.uk	National helpline
Care Standards Authorities As Guide 4	Report any complaints to them

At a Glance – Sheltered Accommodation

- Get an assessment to determine level of care needed
- What can your parents afford?
- Take financial advice
- Go into schemes in detail – what are you paying for/hidden extras etc.

At a Glance – Care Homes

- Get a care assessment
- Discuss it with your parents
- Where do they want to live?
- Check homes in person
- Ask a lot of questions
- Read Care Homes Inspectorate reports
- Keep an eye on local authority financial assessment
- Help your parents to adjust
- Be patient

At a Glance – Moving In With You

- Before you say yes, discuss it with your family
- Get the financial details out into the open with the *whole* family
- Establish ground rules – for you and your parents
- What will happen if their health deteriorates? Discuss it now

Chapter 5

HOSPITAL STAYS

When we're young we take our body for granted – of course
it's bendy, of course we can touch our toes, sit cross-legged on
the floor, run around a football field or tennis court. We throw
ourselves into the sea or the pool with abandon, jump on a
bike, dash for a bus, assuming everything will work perfectly – why shouldn't it?

And in these days of health awareness we can make that
assumption for longer than ever before. There have never been
so many 70-plus marathon runners, scuba divers, scratch
golfers, lap swimmers. We all know the benefits of good nutri-
tion and exercise; we've discovered the Fountain of Youth.
It's fabulous.

But, eventually and inevitably, things start to get creaky. It
happens so gradually we might not notice that it's been a
while since we last bent down without breathing hard, or ran
anywhere, or sat back on our heels. Insidiously, our style is
being cramped.

The next thing we know our GP is prescribing tablets –
something to keep our blood pressure down, maybe a pill to
lower cholesterol. We take it in our stride; that famous ability
to block off mortality kicks in. After all, modern medication
works miracles. We have nothing to worry about.

Your parents might have been taking pills like this for years – for so long it's become the norm – so when parts finally do start wearing out it comes as a bolt from the blue. Maybe it's a broken hip, a prostate problem, a heart attack; whatever it is, it's going to shock them rigid. However many changes they've already had to cope with, a hospital stay at this time in their lives is going to be traumatic.

Quite apart from the illness itself, there's the whole concept of being in hospital and the loss of control that this involves. You're not dressed; you're stuck in a bed, probably several floors up, at the mercy of people who come and go seemingly arbitrarily, and *you can't get out*. It's as if someone has pressed the pause button on your life.

It's upsetting for the family too. You hate to see your parents suffering and helpless, to have to walk away and leave them there, among strangers. Nothing can turn a stay in hospital into a truly pleasant experience, but your understanding and support can help make it as bearable and beneficial as possible.

Dealing with the Idea

The circumstances surrounding your parent's admission can have a profound effect on how they cope with the reality of life on a hospital ward.

Scheduled admittance

If the stay has been planned in advance – a hip replacement, for example – there's an opportunity to help them get into the right frame of mind. They'll have time to discuss with their GP (and hopefully consultant) what's going to be involved, roughly how long they'll be in hospital, what they can expect in terms of recovery time and so on. Knowledge is power and they'll feel much more relaxed and in control if they're fully informed.

You could help them draw up a list of questions to take with them when they go to see the doctor. We're all apt to forget what we wanted to ask until it's too late and, if you're elderly and not very well, things are even more likely to slip your mind.

They might like you to go with them, especially if they have no partner. You don't necessarily have to be present at the actual consultation, but if you're waiting outside they can tell you all about it straight away and any practical queries you might think of could well be tackled on the spot either by asking the nursing/administrative staff or, in the case of medical questions, maybe by leaving a note for the doctor.

In the case of couples, the one who's going into hospital, apart from being worried about themselves, will be concerned about the partner they're leaving behind – can they manage without me? And the one left at home is bound to be wondering the same thing. Elderly couples cope as a team and one can be much less than half as efficient as both together.

The prospect of their partner disappearing into hospital can be a big physical and mental setback, even to the point of panic. It's worth looking at whether they'll need outside help. Depending on their situation and the local authority's rules, this may be forthcoming from social services – and as with all personal care it may or may not be free or part-funded.

In any case, unless they're very fit indeed, they'll need an eye keeping on them while they're on their own. Whoever is going to do this – family, neighbours – it's worth setting up a firm plan and making sure your parents are involved in this and know exactly what's going to be happening.

Planning ahead will help put their mind at rest, and freedom from anxiety can make a pronounced difference to recovery after an illness or an operation.

Emergency admission

Clanging ambulance bells, paramedics, life-support machines – it's very scary for everyone, and for your parents it can be absolutely terrifying. There's no way to prepare for this; it has to be dealt with as it unfolds, but all the normal hospital worries come into force with knobs on.

Try to stay calm and establish a relationship with the appropriate doctor and the nurses.

After the initial dramas of A&E, patients are often sent to some kind of reception ward where their needs are assessed, maybe tests done, and decisions made about which ward they'll be admitted to. These transit wards are essential for preliminary diagnosis, but they're appalling places to be. They're noisy, full of bustling nurses who don't know your name, porters squeezing trolleys with recumbent bodies into tiny spaces, beeping machinery and stressed-out families with bags of clothes and emergency rations. They can feel like a cross between an airport departure lounge and a refugee camp.

This environment is absolutely not conducive to reasoned thinking or calm acceptance. If your parent is conscious and aware of what's going on, they're likely to panic – it's a truly alien world. They need your reassurance and in order to give it to them it's important to get on top of what's going on.

Nurses will be frantically busy, but steel yourself – you need to catch one on the wing and get the story.

There may not actually *be* a story yet of course, and almost certainly no definitive answers, but they can give you some kind of picture of what's happening – when they expect the consultant to appear, how long (roughly) before a move to a regular ward. Whatever scraps of information you glean can be passed on to your parents. They'll be grateful for every crumb.

Of course the hospital will want to move patients out of there and into a specialist ward as quickly as possible, both to make room for someone else and so appropriate treatment can begin, but sometimes the stay in a transit ward can be longer than you'd expect – even days.

There can be a variety of reasons for this. Maybe the diagnosis isn't straightforward; maybe the necessary doctor is doing something else somewhere else, maybe they're waiting for X-rays, or tests are taking a while. Or maybe there just isn't a vacant bed in the right ward – a situation where patients can end up being parked in corridors.

Paula's 80-year-old father Everard had a stroke and was rushed to hospital.

'Dad was left on a trolley out in the hall. He was very ill, but conscious, and terrified. He kept saying, "Get me out of here." He was out of his mind with fear. Mum was hysterical. They just left him where he was, and then he had a second stroke. He never spoke again.'

If your parent is left out in the corridor, start by approaching the nearest nurse and asking why – are they on their way for a test? Is it just for a few minutes? If they're waiting for a ward, how long will it be? Are they just making the bed? Or isn't there one available yet? If it's the latter, or you don't get any answers, insist on speaking to a staff nurse or sister. Be reasonable, measured – but don't be fobbed off. They *will* know if there isn't a bed available – they just might not want to tell you.

If it does look as though your loved one will be spending more than a couple of hours in a corridor, raise hell – in a nice way of course – but be persistent. This is an absolutely unacceptable situation and you need to be very firm.

Quietly insist on your parent being moved, maybe into a side ward for the night, or back to the admissions ward. Try not to get angry or shout, although this is easier said than done. If you're stressed and worried, the temptation to let off steam at *somebody* can be overwhelming. But remember – it isn't the nurses' fault. They aren't in control of bed spaces and they're doing their best in very difficult circumstances. The last thing they need is a family member raging away at them. If you don't get things resolved satisfactorily make a formal complaint.

While They're in Hospital

Hospitals can feel like the last place you want to be ill in. For a start they're horribly intimate. You're lying there in your night things or a hospital gown with inadequate fastenings, looking and feeling your absolute worst just a couple of feet away from a perfect stranger – very often of the opposite sex – in *their* night things. Other semi-clothed strangers are all around you.

Why the NHS feels mixed-sex wards are in any way compatible with human dignity is beyond understanding. Nobody can find them comfortable, but if you're elderly they're a sophisticated form of torture.

To be too unwell to adjust the neck of your nightgown or the front of your pyjama trousers is mortifying for a generation brought up to believe in modesty and privacy. To have to call a nurse for a bedpan or a commode and then sit behind a flimsy curtain within earshot – and smelling distance – of a dozen or so other people is humiliating.

'I was sitting on a commode with my pyjamas round my ankles, but the curtains hadn't closed properly and the lady opposite could see me. I felt ashamed' – Ali, aged 84

In theory, mixed sex wards are now supposed to contain single sex 'bays', but since these are usually screened merely by curtains, the difference is semantic rather than real.

Hospitals save lives, but the wards themselves are rather like town centres – there's a lot of traffic so it's hard to relax. And you're so helpless. The ward routine seems to have nothing to do with you as an individual. Doctors come and go to their own schedule. Just when you've managed to doze off nurses wake you to make your bed, or take your blood pressure or temperature. The evening medicine trolley can make its appearance so late that you're already fast asleep (even with all the ward lights blazing) and need to be woken up again.

It all seems to be an inevitable part of the hospital system. It's not really that staff don't care; they do a truly amazing job in very difficult circumstances. But if you're used to living quietly, the whole atmosphere is unsettling.

Add to this the stress and anxiety of being elderly and ill and you have a recipe for misery. It's not surprising your parent can become depressed if the stay is anything other than short.

The thing to remember above all is that your parent will be afraid; afraid of what the illness itself will do to them; afraid they'll never come out of hospital – that they'll die there; afraid that if they do get out they'll be packed off to a care home; afraid of what's happening to their partner in their absence.

Sometimes this overall fear will fix itself on just one aspect of the situation and blow it up out of all proportion.

Kevin's mother Louise was 85 when she went into hospital after a slight stroke.

'All she worried about was Dad – she couldn't believe that he was OK. He was living at home with some help from a neighbour and doing fine, but she seemed to think we were neglecting him. We'd take him in to see her and try to reason with her but she'd get all het up and shout at us, saying we had to sell our house and move to look after Dad. He was wonderful with her – the only one who could calm her down.

'She'd go on and on to the nurses about how there was nobody to care for him, and demand to go home. It was a great hospital and the staff were super – they explained to us what was making Mum act irrationally, that it was partly fear and partly the results of the stroke.'

It would have been easy for Kevin and his family to get angry with Louise, and defensive about why they weren't looking after him themselves, but because of what the nurses had said they understood what was happening and tried to be patient.

A hospital stay is just as frightening for the partner left behind. Zeb's wife Tricia went into hospital for tests, and was kept there for three months. Their son Andrew took Zeb home with him, but he lived 250 miles from the hospital.

'At first it was fine, Dad settled in happily. He was worried about Mum of course – we all were, but we'd take Dad to visit her every couple of weeks and they'd talk on the phone.

'Then as time went on he started to worry about why she wasn't coming out. He kept asking us if we were keeping something from him. We kept trying to explain but he didn't believe us.

'He started eavesdropping on our phone conversations. We'd be talking to someone completely unconnected with Mum, and he'd pick up an extension and demand to know what was going on.'

'If he'd been able to see her more often it might not have been so bad, but it got to the point where he was pining so much we had to move him back home. Social services assessed him and gave him some temporary help until Mum came home.'

Zeb was terrified he was being kept out of the loop and needed the reassurance of seeing his wife. She, on the other hand, was happier knowing he was safe with the family. If circumstances allow, try to talk through the pros and cons of the various options beforehand with them both, so they can decide what arrangement they'd prefer.

Sometimes you might not be completely happy with the care your parent is receiving. It's a sad fact that some hospitals are better than others and, on top of that, many hospital wards these days tend to have a preponderance of patients with dementia, which puts a different kind of pressure on nursing staff and patients alike.

David's 90-year-old mother Zoe had a fall and was admitted to a large hospital.

'Mum didn't have a window and there was nobody for her to talk to because none of the other patients could hold a lucid conversation. As a result she didn't get any mental stimulation at all.

'The staff never had time to get Mum out of bed, although she was supposed to have short walks as part of her treatment, and she only got physiotherapy once a week.'

'They put her on a catheter, even though she could have walked to the toilet with help – and she wanted to. Was it because they were so busy they were trying to cut down on jobs? She went downhill both physically and mentally during the ten weeks she was in that hospital. I felt cruel leaving her there.'

If you're unhappy, talk to the ward sister and explain your worries. This should be enough to clear things up but if it doesn't, there are complaints procedures. Don't be afraid that if you complain the staff will take it out on your parent – nurses are compassionate people; they're overworked, not ogres.

It's important to keep up your parent's morale. Visiting times will be just about all they have to look forward to. There's nothing more likely to bring on a bout of self-pity than watching everyone else's visitors when you don't have any of your own. If you can't get there as often as you'd like, try to organize a rota with their friends and the rest of the family – this is another of those fraught areas where one person can end up taking all the strain. If your parents are members of a church or club, alert the vicar or the club secretary, they'll be happy to organize visits too.

There are other ways you can cheer them up, perhaps by bringing in little treats – small helpings of meals you know they like (hospital food is rarely tempting). But check on their diet before you do this. Taking them along for a snack in the hospital café or to the foyer shop for a browse can work wonders too.

If they're well enough it can help enormously to take them out into the fresh air for a while. Even the sight of the car park will be a refreshing change – it's a glimpse of normal life.

Getting the full picture

You'll try to keep your anxieties at bay for your parents' sake, but your own morale is likely to be suffering too. Not knowing what's happening can contribute heavily to your parents' fear factor and destroy your own peace of mind, but getting information can be hard – the system isn't geared up for it.

Most doctors and nurses will explain things to their patients – in fact they're legally obliged to – but depending how ill they are your parents might not remember much, or be confused about who said what and when. This means it will fall to you to find out what's going on.

The trouble is, to an outsider there doesn't seem to be much continuity. Nursing staff work complex shift patterns and on top of that can be moved around to fill needs in different wards – there just aren't enough nurses to go round. Even if you visited at the same time every day you wouldn't necessarily encounter the same nurses very often.

So it's quite possible that the nurse you approach for information won't be familiar with the case, or will only just have come on duty and won't have an update for you. In any case, they're not supposed to give out much information, especially the more junior staff.

Your best bet is to catch the staff nurse or the ward sister. This can be harder than it looks, but there'll be a nurse's station on the ward and you can ask whoever is currently manning it for the person you want.

Senior nurses have the experience to use their own discretion about what they tell, and to whom. They're very knowledgeable and, if you're worried, five minutes with them can help a lot, even if the news isn't very good.

If you live a long distance away or can't get in to see them often, phone the ward and ask for the staff nurse or sister specifically. They're unlikely to discuss diagnosis, but they will tell you how your parent is going on from day to day, their state of mind, when they're seeing the doctor and so on.

Doctors, on the other hand, are something else entirely. They tend to be extremely elusive and tracking one down can be a major undertaking.

Jean's father, 90-year-old Ewan, was in a hospital three hours' drive away.

'Dad was pretty ill. We couldn't get up to see him every day, but between us my brother and I got there about once a week. Sometimes he'd be asleep for the whole visit, at other times he'd be awake but wouldn't really know what was happening.

'My brother and I both spent ages on the phone trying to get hold of Dad's doctor. We'd phone the ward and leave messages asking him to call. Then days later the registrar might ring us, or a junior doctor, or if we were very lucky, the consultant, but we never got the same person twice and they all had a slightly different perspective. Sometimes they seemed to be contradicting each other – it was maddening.'

Jean's experience is very common. Doctors don't mean to be unhelpful, but they can lack imagination. They dash between wards, patients and emergencies, possibly not giving a high priority to the follow-up call you're waiting for so anxiously. And with older patients, several factors may be affecting their condition, which can mean involving various specialists. Given that they all have individual timetables, locating them can be fantastically difficult as they zoom from hospital to hospital. What's more, they'll each be dealing with different aspects of your parent's condition and so might not feel they can comment on the big picture.

Ask the ward sister for the name of the consultant in over-all charge of the case, and get their secretary's phone number. It's very likely they won't be based at that hospital, but the secretary will know all their movements and can try to make sure they ring you, or give you an appointment for a chat.

Most doctors realize the importance of keeping families of elderly patients informed, and should be prepared to make themselves available to you. It doesn't always happen, how-ever. Not all doctors are good at communicating, as Lisa found when her 80-year-old mother Edna was in hospital.

'Mum was in hospital for eight weeks and until right at the end we never saw her consultant.'

'He wouldn't make a specific appointment to see us and we were told to wait for him outside the ward after he'd finished his rounds. Several times my husband took whole days off work to do this, but though we'd sometimes see the doctor in the distance, we didn't manage to catch him.

'We were frantic with worry about Mum, and none of her doctors seemed prepared to take the time to explain things to us. We felt completely impotent – it was like banging your head against a brick wall. One day we finally flagged the consultant down and he looked very put out about it. He wanted to talk to us there in the corridor! We put our foot down and insisted we go somewhere more private.'

If you have trouble chasing up a consultant by phone, try sending an email with your questions via his secretary. Explain that you're worried and why, and ask for an appointment.

Getting Ready for Discharge

From the moment you go into hospital you're focused on getting out again. This is especially true for elderly patients because the limbo that is hospital is so difficult for them to come to terms with. Discharge is the dream . . .

As your parent starts to recover, someone on the hospital staff, along with social services, should be looking at their capabilities with a view to working out what will need to happen when they leave.

This is called the Single Assessment Process (in Scotland it's a Single Shared Assessment Process). It's essentially the same as the assessment covered in Chapters 2 and 3, but co-ordinated by the hospital. What it means is that everyone involved – doctors, nurses, the local authority (maybe the housing department for example), social services, occupational therapists – combines forces to explore whether the patient can be discharged to their own home and with what help, or whether they'll need residential care, and what kind.

The hospital then has to make sure everything necessary, whatever it is, from meals on wheels to personal care to a place in a care home, is set up and ready before they go home.

If your parent is in a private hospital they're still entitled to a free assessment, but they'll probably have to alert the local authority themselves, or you can do it on their behalf. Once the assessment is complete, the rules about who pays for what are the same as for any other kind of personal or residential care (see guides at the end of Chapters 2, 3 and 4).

This is also a time when continuing NHS care can become an issue. The NHS assessment should take place first, and it's appropriate to ask for one if you think your parent might qualify (see Chapter 4).

It might be difficult for the hospital to predict exactly when your parent is going to be discharged – their condition could vary, and doctors shouldn't release them until it's absolutely certain they're stable. Sometimes a period of rehabilitation might be recommended (the NHS should pay for any health care needed). The rehabilitation might take the form of some extra help at home for a while – anything from physiotherapy to prescription collection – or a stay in a different hospital. It will depend on local practice and, of course, the state of your parent's health. But any delay can be very hard for your parent to accept, and they'll worry – is there something they're not telling me?

Lydia's mother Minnie was 82 when she went into hospital with suspected cancer.

'They did a lot of tests, which were very tiring in themselves, and she found the whole experience exhausting. The staff were fantastic and really looked after Mum but she couldn't settle down.

'Naturally, after her operation they wouldn't discharge her until she was ready and they kept putting back the date. She just kept asking – when am I going home? It was all she could think about.'

The longer they kept Minnie the more afraid she became that she'd never get out, and she began to fret. This became so pronounced that Lydia approached the ward sister and they both sat down with Minnie and talked her through what was happening.

They explained that she was still rather wobbly and they wanted to make absolutely sure she could cope when she went home; they reassured her she *would* be going home, and said she could help to get herself better by not worrying so much. Lydia could have done this alone, but she knew that although her mother trusted her, the ward sister would carry more weight.

Of course you don't want your parent to be discharged until they're ready, but sometimes the delay can be *too* long. Ava's father Bruce was in hospital for several weeks after a fall.

'Dad was 84 and had been very well until then, but the hospital seemed to knock him right back. It was a huge place and not very efficient. Nobody seemed to know how to deal with people and I don't think Dad was treated like a human being.

'He was supposed to be moving to the local cottage hospital for some rehab, but the doctors didn't seem to agree on his assessment and it just went on and on. We couldn't get a decision but we didn't want to get cross and antagonize them.'

'When Dad was finally moved he was beyond rehab really, and he died in the cottage hospital just two weeks after going there. Our consolation is that at least he was treated with dignity there. They were very kind and caring.'

The delay could have been simply because it was difficult for Bruce's doctors to decide what would be best for him, but it's understandable for Ava to feel things could have been handled better, because nobody took the time to talk to her about it.

Anita feels her father Douglas was treated in the opposite way, and pushed out of hospital before he was ready.

'Dad was 81 and had a mild stroke. He didn't get out of what they called the medical assessment unit – the reception ward – for over a week because there wasn't room for him on the stroke ward. It was packed. It took a few weeks but he did eventually pull round. Then suddenly they said he could go home. He didn't seem very well to us but we aren't experts, and naturally Dad was desperate to leave.

'We took him home and within hours he'd had another stroke and was rushed back to hospital in an ambulance. I don't think they should ever have discharged him in the first place.'

If you're concerned your parent is being discharged too soon, have a word with the ward sister or the doctor. If you're still worried, ask for a second opinion.

Going Back Home

If it's looking likely that your parent will be able to go back to their own home, the hospital may take them there for a few hours to see how they get on. Then any modifications needed – even door widening for a wheelchair – can be made before they leave hospital. This sounds fine, but although all hospitals should have some kind of single assessment process, they each have their own methods, and aren't necessarily all equally efficient at implementing them.

Robin's 82-year-old mother, Cecily, was due to be discharged from hospital.

'She'd had a couple of mini strokes and was rather weak but the doctors said she should be able to cope, with help. The hospital social worker and an occupational therapist took her on a home visit to see how she'd handle it and they told us she'd need someone to help her in and out of bed.

'But when I rang the local social services to discuss what the hospital had said, they didn't know anything about it. I ended up explaining to *them* what had been decided. They'd obviously never talked to each other at all.'

This lack of communication can mean things don't get done, services don't get put in place and, worst of all for your parents, discharge can be delayed. Talk to the hospital social worker or your parent's case manager if you're concerned things aren't happening as they should.

Discussing arrangements with your parent will keep them positive and give them something to look forward to. Apart from the direct effects of the illness itself, the whole experience might have left them psychologically less able to cope than before, and these chats will give them the chance to voice any fears.

They might have made a good recovery, but lying in a hospital bed for several weeks – perhaps even months – can result in a disconnection from reality. They've been out of the world for so long it can seem like waking up after being in suspended animation, and things they'd normally do without thinking can seem beyond them. They'll be physically weak too – their muscle tone will have gone after all that sitting and lying about.

Even if they aren't going to need any significant help it can be very reassuring for them to know well in advance who's going to be taking them home, and that someone will be giving their house a tidy-up, getting it warm and doing some shopping. Talk to the rest of the family about it – there's no reason why it should all be done by one person. There are charities that help in these situations too.

Ask social services if they'll keep an eye on your parent for a couple of weeks after they leave hospital, especially if you don't live nearby.

It's helpful to ask the hospital to explain any medication to you before your parent leaves, so you can reinforce what they've been told. They're likely to forget in all the upheaval.

Leaving Hospital for Residential Care

It's possible that the illness has left your parent too frail to go home at all, and they'll need to go straight into a care home or sheltered accommodation. This can feel like a total disaster, a line drawn under their life. Imagine, one minute you're at home as usual, then you're uprooted into the surreal environment of a hospital; perhaps you've been so ill you almost died and you're already having to cope with the fact of disability or great frailty – and now you learn you'll never live in your own home again.

The very idea of this can be enough to produce a relapse. Spend time explaining to your parent why it needs to happen and help them come to terms with it. They'll have plenty of worries (see Chapter 4). Nobody can force your parent into a home, but once they cease to need proper hospital care they won't be allowed to take up a bed indefinitely.

Gertrude was 92 when she had a heart attack and had to go from hospital into a care home.

'I didn't really have a choice. I wasn't well enough to look after myself, but it was hard. The children sorted out

my things. I went back once to look through them but I couldn't stand it, so I told them to get on with it. I've never seen my lovely bungalow since.'

If they're not well enough to visit their home, talk through each room with them, discussing the contents and remembering the stories that go with them – do you remember when you brought back that clock from your holiday in Spain? That way they're more likely to remember the things *they* really want to have around them, and not just what someone else thinks they might like.

Choosing a care home is difficult enough at any time, and it's doubly hard to do when they're still in a hospital bed. For a start they probably won't be able to visit potential homes so you'll need to be their eyes and ears. Sometimes the manager of a prospective home will visit them in hospital so they can ask questions. Help them to draw up a list of issues that matter to them (see Chapter 4).

Who'll pay is assessed exactly as it would be if your parent wasn't in hospital – but if they qualify for fully paid continuing NHS care, they may not get a choice of home. If your parent was already living in a home before going into hospital, even if they were paying for it themselves, it might not be suitable for their changed state of health and they might need to find a different home (see Chapter 4). Maybe the home can provide the extra care but charges more for it. If this is the case and the local authority or NHS is paying all or part of the fees, you may find they won't pay the extra cost – it could be beyond their budget – every area has its own rules (see guides in Chapter 4). This might mean a move, but if there are no places in a cheaper suitable home, then the local authority will have to pay the extra, however reluctant they are. It's worth looking into what local policy is so you can twist a few arms if necessary.

Another difficulty can be when the patient's partner is already in a home. Will it agree to take both of them? Can it provide the right care for both of them? This again might precipitate a move, or the decision that they'll live in different homes.

A similar situation arises if one of your parents is still living at home. Can they continue to do this on a more permanent basis? Do they want to? If so they'll need an assessment.

These are tough questions, and your parents need some time to think about them. The hospital should give them that time, not hustle them into any old home just because there's a place, or because they need the bed.

If the home they've chosen doesn't have a space available then they could go somewhere else temporarily – but make sure the local authority knows it's temporary and they don't get stuck permanently somewhere they don't want to be.

Suzanne's mother Cynthia was in hospital after a stroke, and it became clear she wouldn't be able to look after herself at home.

'Mum was adamant that she wanted to be in one particular home. We all liked it and wanted her to go there. Unfortunately there was a waiting list and she needed to come out of hospital. The local authority was paying her fees and they said she could go to another home temporarily.

'It was an awful place – it didn't smell very nice and there was no garden at all, just a paved yard. The rooms were tiny and scruffy. It reminded me of how youth hostels used to be when I was a kid. Mum hated it, but there didn't seem anything we could do, so we hung on for two or three months.

'I could see she was miserable and was worried that her health would suffer again, so I mentioned it to social services, and asked them how the waiting list was going. It must have jogged their elbow because she got a place in the original home within a few weeks. She's much happier now, but I do wonder what would have happened if I hadn't said anything.'

Suzanne's experience shows how important it is to keep talking to all the agencies involved. It can help prevent your parents from dropping through a hole in the system. And it's a good idea to be well aware of their rights. Local authorities are generally well intentioned, but some are in such straitened financial circumstances they might be tempted to bend the rules – even their own.

The guides overleaf will give you a start on how to help your parent handle a hospital stay.

Guide 1 – Admission to Hospital

Situation	Useful Contacts
Some of your benefits may alter	Disability Benefits Unit: 0845 7123456 Northern Ireland Disability and Carers' Service: 02890 906178 Help the Aged SeniorLine: 0808 8006565 Northern Ireland: 0808 8087575 Citizens' Advice Bureaux (see local phone book)
Carer's benefits might alter	Carer's Allowance Unit: 01253 856123 Northern Ireland 02890 906186 SeniorLine as above

Guide 2 –
Discharge From Hospital to Your Own Home

Situation	Useful Contacts
Single Assessment Process (SAP, or SSAP in Scotland). A co-ordinated team headed by your hospital assesses your care needs. Can include a visit home from hospital.	England/Wales: Social Services Scotland: Social Work Department Northern Ireland: Social Services Trust All numbers in local phone books. Ask for the hospital staff member in charge of your case
Carers can have an assessment too	Local authorities, as above Carers UK: 0808 8087777
Who pays for what?	See chapters 2&3
NHS Continuing Care (NHS funded care) Assessment for this should be done before SAP. Ask for one if you think you might qualify. Very complex criteria and regional interpretations	See Chapter 4 Age Concern has fact sheets Information Line – 0800 009966 www.ace.org.uk Help the Aged SeniorLine (as Guide 1) NHS Helpline for Scotland: 0800 224488
Help preparing your house for your return	Red Cross www.redcross.org.uk Help The Aged Home From Hospital – (See local phone book for numbers)
Having benefits reinstated	Social Security – (see local phone book)
Ask hospital to explain your medicine	Your staff nurse Help The Aged Leaflets SeniorLine, as above

Guide 3 –
Discharge to a Care Home/Sheltered Housing

Situation	Useful Contacts
Single Assessment Process Don't be pushed by the hospital into choosing in a hurry or going somewhere you don't want to go.	As Guide 2
Who pays?	See Chapter 4 and guides
NHS Continuing Care You could be eligible – assessment should be done before SAP	As Guide 2
Choosing a home for you and/or your partner	See Chapter 4 and guides

Guide 4 – Your Rights

Situation	Useful Contacts
Under the Citizens' Charter, as a hospital patient you have various rights, including privacy, respect for your culture, the right to information, and to refuse treatment.	Patients' Charter (part of Citizens' Charter) www.nhs.uk Your hospital social worker Citizens' Advice Bureaux – (see local phone book)
You can query your assessment if you disagree with it	Member of hospital staff in charge of your SAP Your local authority social worker
You should not be pushed into leaving hospital to go home until all your care package is in place	Your SAP manager, as above Citizens' Advice Bureaux – (see local phone book) Social Services – (see local phone book) Age Concern has advice: 0800 009966 www.ace.org.uk Red Cross – (see local phone book) www.redcross.org.uk
You can't be discharged to a care home without your consent	As above
If you're unhappy with your experiences with a doctor or hospital	Patients' Association 0845 6084455 www.patients-association.org.uk

Guide 5 – Making a Complaint

Problem	Contact
Dissatisfaction with your care in hospital	Ward sister Hospital liaison service Ombudsman (Chapter 4, Guide 10)
A complaint about the NHS	England: Independent Complaints Advocacy Service Northern Ireland: Health and Social services Councils – hospital liaison service will have local numbers Scotland: NHS Boards Wales: Community Health Councils SeniorLine: 0808 8006565 (Northern Ireland: 0808 8087575) Citizens' Advice Bureaux – (see local phone book)
Advice on complaints procedures	Citizens' Advice Bureaux – as above

At a Glance

- Contact the Dept of Social Security about their benefits
- Keep in touch with nurses/doctors
- Does the partner remaining behind need any help?
- Organize a visiting rota
- Keep an eye on the assessment
- Check on eligibility for NHS continuing care
- Plan ahead – is their house ready for their discharge?
- Discuss any plans with your parents
- Don't allow them to be sent home until a care package is in place
- Help them come to terms with any changes in their health
- Involve them in any choice of home or sheltered housing
- Don't let them be pushed out of hospital into any old care home

Chapter 6

MENTAL DISORDERS

What makes you *you*? Not the colour of your eyes or the size of your feet; not your height or weight, although these can have a profound effect. What makes you who you are is inside your head – all those electrical impulses sparking away, enabling you to think, feel, reason, react.

Medical science hasn't yet fully fathomed the human brain – it's miraculous, a mystery, our most precious (and least understood) attribute. So of all the things that happen to us as we age, the loss of mental capacity is the most frightening and the most final. Good maintenance – diet and exercise, drugs and surgery – can keep our mechanical parts running smoothly well into old age, but if the circuitry fails there's no getting it back. We can lose our ability to function, our whole personality. And it happens to a lot of us. Over 700,000 people over the age of 65 in the UK have dementia, and by 2050 it's estimated the figure could be approaching 2 million. That's because we're all living longer and, the older we get, the greater our chance of developing it.

It's many people's biggest fear. We don't relish the idea of losing our mobility, sight, hearing, or enduring any of the other lurking incapacities in the catalogue of ageing – but they pale into insignificance before the spectre of dementia.

No surprise, then, that we don't want to recognize the signs, either in ourselves or in those we love; we push aside the very idea as unthinkable. To watch the disintegration of a personality, to experience the disintegration of your own, is a dreadful cruelty.

Of all the things we have to come to terms with as our parents age, dementia must be the hardest. It can provoke a whole range of violent emotions in them and in us – everything from straight denial to anger and fear. Sucked into a black hole of unrelieved misery, anxiety and hard work, we can find it impossible to deal with. Families can be split apart. Death can seem like a light at the end of the tunnel.

Don't feel guilty and blame yourself or your parents for feelings that neither you nor they can help. Instead, try to understand what they're going through, and your own reactions to it. Cut yourself some slack and you'll make it easier for them too. Don't be hard on yourself and you'll be less inclined to be hard on them.

Am I Losing My Mind?

By far the most common form of dementia is Alzheimer's disease, followed by vascular dementia, which is caused by damaged blood vessels, for example when someone has a stroke.

There are other kinds too, but whatever type it is, the early signs can be hard to spot because they're the kind of thing everyone's liable to on a bad day – particularly forgetfulness. We dismiss our parents' memory lapses as a normal part of growing older, and in most cases they're just that – and of course we have them too. Senior moments are a joke, so why should we take them seriously?

And you might not worry unduly if they have the odd

moment of confusion or hesitation in making a decision. You tell yourself they're just getting on a bit; there's nothing really wrong.

Katherine's parents Madeleine and Roland were in their late seventies when Madeleine had a thrombosis.

'She seemed all right afterwards, but looking back that must have been when her dementia first started. At first, all we noticed was that Mum became very dependent on Dad. She clung to him all the time, as though she felt she could cope better physically when he wasn't out of sight.

'Mum slowly got more absent-minded and less capable but we left them alone, thinking "if it isn't broke, don't fix it". You want your parents to be the way you've always known them.

'I used to be quite short with Mum. It was almost cruel. I'd tell her to pull herself together – that of course she could manage. I'd stop her from running to Dad for help, and make her do things for herself. I kept hoping she'd agree with me that she *was* being silly so that I could be wrong about her having a problem. But in the back of my mind I knew . . .'

'Then they went on a cruise and when they came back Dad told me that Mum had been much worse – people had been embarrassed by her behaviour. He asked me what I thought and I suppose at that point I began to face it.'

Katherine feels guilty about the way she tried to jolly her mother along, but it was her way of denying anything was wrong. Her behaviour came from love and respect for the person Madeleine had been. It's hard to do, but it might have been better if she'd tried to accept what was happening to Madeleine rather than hanging on to the past.

When your parents try to hide the situation it can be even

tougher to spot. Joanna's mother Carrie started to lose her short-term memory when she was 90.

'Mum was as fit as a fiddle, but she'd been widowed for 25 years and had never really got over losing my dad. She'd become a bit of a stranger to the truth, to be honest, and we were used to that, so we didn't realize she was starting Alzheimer's disease.

'She wouldn't admit that her memory was wobbly, and she developed strategies to deal with it and cover it up. We'd tell her something and she'd ask the next person who came to visit to write it down for her. Then she'd forget again, and end up with a stack of notes. Even much later, when she got to the stage where she didn't know what day it was, she'd deny that anything was wrong.'

It's likely that at first Carrie genuinely didn't notice her memory lapses. When she did start to suspect, her first reaction would naturally have been to deny it to herself and to her family, so although Joanna was very close to her mother, it's not surprising she and her husband didn't notice a problem – Carrie was doing everything she could to make sure they didn't.

And who can blame her? After all, given how tempted we are to ignore even minor signs of ageing (see Chapters 2 and 3), how much more likely is it that we'd brush aside any hint that we might be 'losing it'?

Whatever form it takes, dementia is incurable and progressive, although some of the symptoms can be treated. Symptoms vary widely, but they gradually become much harder to miss, like forgetting how to do physical things like get dressed or eat properly.

As with other problems, if you don't see your parents all that often – if you live a long distance away for example – it can be even more difficult to pick up on. Grant's father Murdoe had lived alone for many years.

'Dad was 81 when we first noticed that he was becoming forgetful. We'd phone a couple of times a week and we started to realize he was telling us all the things he'd told us just two or three days before, and asking questions we'd already answered.

'On our trips to see him he was more or less the same as usual and for several months we told ourselves we were imagining things. Then one weekend we were chatting to his neighbour, and she mentioned that he'd been locking himself out of the house quite a lot. She had a key and had been able to let him in, but she said he'd been "rather vague".

'I asked Dad about it and he seemed normal enough. He told me there was something wrong with the lock and asked me to fix it, but when I had a look it was fine. I asked him to lock and unlock the door for me and I could see that he wasn't putting in the key properly. I showed him over and over again how to do it, but he kept on locking himself out. And every time we spoke he'd ask me to mend it as if he'd never mentioned it before.

'Then we'd arrive to find plates of half-eaten dinner on the lawn, and the house began to be a mess. He was losing touch with reality and we knew we'd have to do something before he hurt himself.'

Grant talked to Murdoe's doctor, who diagnosed Alzheimer's disease. Some personal care was arranged for him and he was able to continue living at home for quite a while, although eventually he couldn't look after himself and agreed to go into a care home.

If you begin to suspect something might be wrong, try to get your parent to see their GP, who can arrange an assessment to work out what, if any, support is needed (see Chapters 2 and 3).

The same principles apply as with any kind of age-related infirmity, except the experts will probably now include a psychiatrist and maybe a continence adviser. The latter will look closely at your parent's condition and decide whether continence pads are required and if so what kind – there are dozens of types. These are delivered on a regular basis and should, unless they're only needed for a very short time, be free.

Even doctors can have a hard time recognizing the signs of dementia. There are no clear-cut tests and the symptoms can be confused with other things – bereavement, stress or anxiety about a partner. It's also possible to have more than one kind of dementia at the same time. What's more, some medical conditions have very similar symptoms, so it could actually be something else altogether – something treatable, maybe curable, like an infection. That's why it's important to try for a diagnosis as early as possible.

There are tests to check on short-term memory loss, but they aren't always conclusive, as Alec found with his father Keith.

'Dad was 85 and had been getting steadily more forgetful. Mum's been unwell for a long time and she has a memory problem too, so he was used to being the strong one. He kept saying that he was fine, but Mum pushed him into going to see his GP.

'The doctor asked him simple questions like his date of birth and address, and he did OK with these. Then he mentioned three things – an apple, a banana and a pear, and asked Dad to repeat them. He got them all right but a few minutes later, when the doctor asked him again what they were, he couldn't remember. He kept going back to it, but Dad never got them right again.

'The doctor asked Dad how he felt. He said, "I've never been 85 before – I don't know what it *should* feel like".'

Keith hasn't been given any help, and what worries Alec is that his father doesn't know there's anything wrong with him. And why should he? The symptoms can come and go. What's very clear to you because you know your parents so well can be hard for a doctor to diagnose in just a couple of sessions.

Melanie's father Eddie was in his early eighties when his wife had a hip operation.

'Dad seemed to go downhill as soon as Mum went into hospital. I went to stay with them when she came home and he'd gone to pieces – he couldn't even make a sandwich. He kept asking me what was wrong with Mum, repeating himself. Yet sometimes he was absolutely fine.

'We made him see the doctor, who said that although he's got some short-term memory loss he's as good as he was five years ago. It's claptrap. Half the time Dad doesn't even know what day it is or what he's had for dinner.'

It might surprise you to find that even if your parent is diagnosed as having dementia, if it's in the early stages they might be assessed as not needing any assistance. This can be for several reasons. It's thought that having as normal a life as possible, with things to challenge them and make them think, can sometimes help to slow the advance of dementia. On the other hand, if the local authority is strapped for resources, they might use this as an excuse and say your parent 'isn't bad enough' to need help.

If you don't agree with your parent's doctor or the local authority assessment, and you don't believe they're capable of managing alone, talk to the social services department and ask them to take another look. Your parent is entitled to be reassessed, but of course they themselves might not *want* to disagree with an assessment that says they're OK. Explain the situation to the social worker and ask for advice.

A dramatic event like the death of a partner can coincide with such a downturn that what you might only have suspected before becomes frighteningly clear. Shirley had been suffering from some memory loss and confusion for a while, but it was only when her husband Malcolm died that their daughter Sandra realized her mother had dementia.

'Mum had been just about managing but I think Dad had been doing most things. Then he had a heart attack and died within an hour.

'When I arrived Mum was completely lucid and coping beautifully. She even told me that Dad wouldn't have wanted me to cry. It was as though she was acting a part. I don't think she'd grasped that Dad was dead. Then when it hit her the following day she was hysterical.

'At the funeral I don't think she even realized it was for Dad and I didn't tell her. I didn't want other people to know the mental state she was in. I wanted to save her face.'

The pity Sandra felt for her mother is perfectly natural, but it's often just what your parents want to avoid. Fear of pity is one of the reasons they conceal what's going on.

Coping as a Couple

It's desperately sad watching someone you love struggling with dementia. If one of your parents has a problem, the other will be going through hell. The dynamics of their relationship will shift, fall out of balance – a previously solid partnership can become fragile for the first time.

The partner who's well is going to hide their suspicions for as long as possible. If it were you what would you do? For a start you wouldn't want to believe it, and if you did finally face it, what then? Do you tell your children, 'I think your dad/mum is losing it a bit'? How disloyal would that feel? And what if your partner found out what you were saying – they'd feel completely betrayed.

You might feel ashamed too – there's still so much stigma attached to mental illness. It's absolutely instinctive to keep any doubts to yourself and try to carry on normally.

Wendy's mother Dolly tried to do just that when her husband Roger started having problems.

'Mum and Dad were both 80 and seemed to be doing so well for their age. Then Mum began to be snappy with me – something she'd never done. One day she just burst into tears and I sat her down and asked what was wrong. She told me Dad had been having "funny turns". He'd go off into a trance for a few minutes then he'd come round, but after each one he seemed a bit more vague. It was terrifying her.

'We'd been joking with Dad that he was forgetting things but we'd had no idea about this. Mum had just bottled it all up. Dad saw the doctor, who said he thought he'd been having a series of mini strokes. He put Dad on some medication and the strokes have stopped. He's a lot better physically but his short-term memory is very patchy. Mum's dealing with it better now she knows what's wrong.'

What had been frightening Dolly, quite apart from seeing her husband like this, was the responsibility of deciding whether or not to call the doctor when Roger was having an attack. He always recovered in a few minutes and she knew he'd be cross if she made a fuss, but she could see the changes in him and they worried her. Getting to the bottom of it meant she had guidelines – the doctor had told her how to react, so she felt more secure and in control.

Even when someone has been diagnosed as having a problem it doesn't mean they're going to admit it or accept it, and this makes it harder still for the partner who's doing the caring.

Mona's mother Ruth went to see their GP herself when she realized her husband Tony's memory was deteriorating. The doctor saw him and said he wasn't bad enough to need help.

'It's awful for Mum seeing Dad like this every day, and he doesn't make it any easier. He gets mad if it's mentioned, won't discuss it or acknowledge that there's anything wrong at all, and it really gets Mum down. And he's still driving his car, which frightens us all.'

'Dad's exasperated by paperwork – anything to do with bills and so on – because he can't understand it. He can't keep up so he ducks out and just eats, sleeps, sits about and reads the paper.

'Mum's a proud woman and doesn't find it easy to talk about private things, but now she phones me every day and cries – she has to let it out to somebody. She doesn't want Dad to know she's phoning me. She's in a vacuum.

'I'm not in their everyday lives because they live miles away, and I try to see things from the doctor's point of view, but Mum's so stressed – she has panic attacks, and it's all down to her worries about Dad.'

It would be easy for Mona to blame her father for his attitude as she watches her mother suffering – and that's exactly what can happen where families watch one parent bearing the brunt of the other's dementia.

But from Tony's point of view his behaviour makes perfect

sense. If *you* found yourself unable to fathom everyday things like opening the post; if you sometimes couldn't remember what you had for lunch or how to tie your shoelaces, you'd get angry – with yourself first and foremost – and then at anyone who presumed to point it out to you; even if they loved you; even if they were on your side and trying to help. You wouldn't want it to be true, so you'd reject the whole idea.

What must it be like to know there are times when you're not completely lucid, when you might do or say things that aren't 'normal'. You'd spend the whole time you're OK dreading the times when you weren't. You'd be absolutely terrified.

Try to imagine how that feels before you jump on a parent who seems to be acting unreasonably or getting cross. Remember too that irritability can be part of the dementia itself, and as much out of your parent's control as getting spots when you have measles.

And it cuts the other way. The partner who's doing the caring can become angry and bitter. Max's parents Edgar and Genevieve are in their eighties and live at home together.

'Mum had a couple of minor strokes eight or nine years ago and began to lose her short-term memory and her ability to do everyday tasks. Dad has looked after her for a long time and he still thinks he's managing – but he's not. He makes lists every morning and tries to keep everything together, but it's nearly lunchtime before he gets going.

'He puts a lot of pressure on Mum. He gets cross with her when she forgets and asks him the same question a hundred times. Then she gets flustered and it makes her worse.'

You can see why Edgar gets angry. He hates to see Genevieve struggling to cope with ordinary everyday things, so he gets impatient, tells her to snap out of it, to try harder. It would be better if Edgar could encourage rather than criticize, to give Genevieve confidence in herself. If joined-up jobs like setting the table are too much, splitting them into small parts might work. So instead of asking her to set the table and getting cross when she makes a hash of it, he could suggest getting the forks out of the drawer, then when she's managed that, ask her to lay them on the table and so on.

It's hard to face, but in fact it's better to regard the whole process as being like teaching a young child – you give praise and encouragement when they get it right, but you try not to patronize them.

Debbie's father Terry had a different way of dealing with his wife Margaret's dementia.

'Mum's short-term memory was going but she could still hold a normal conversation and Dad behaved as if she was OK.

'When Mum was vague in front of people he'd pretend it was just absence of mind and tell her to be more up to date, to read the papers. It did sound patronizing, but he was protecting her. You don't want people to think your wife has a mental problem and judge her by that, do you?'

What Terry was experiencing was another form of denial, a natural response to the heartbreak of watching someone you love gradually lose their dignity – and dignity is a very precious thing. Michaela and Carl are both in their late eighties and Carl has severe Alzheimer's disease.

Carl doesn't recognize his wife of over sixty years. But she has her standards. She knows how much store her husband always set by being well dressed, so every day she makes sure he's wearing a smart collar and tie. He doesn't remember how he used to be, but she does.

All the problems of being a carer for your partner are multiplied a thousandfold when they have dementia. As it progresses it can strip away all vestiges of the person you knew. The partner with whom you've raised children and shared a whole lifetime of experiences, whom you still love most in the world, doesn't know your name or recognize your face.

The person you've relied on to be there for you through all life's ups and downs can't put a coherent thought together. Their body is present, but their mind is gone. What you suffer, seeing this, is grief. You're as bereft as if your partner had died – maybe more so.

Dementia can bring with it the inability to form words and perform the simplest tasks. Your partner might wet the bed because they've forgotten to go to the toilet, or suddenly think that a rubbish bin in the street is the loo and start to use it; they can spend the night walking about looking for something they mislaid on their wedding day; they might see things that aren't there. And with the best will in the world, a lot of their habits are quite simply annoying – they get to you.

So it's easy for a carer to become bitter – why is this happening to us? And it's a very lonely job. You might not want other people to see your partner in this state; you could be afraid to go out and leave them alone in case they scald themselves or fall down the stairs. And there's no end to it, no way out.

It can be a big relief to have someone to talk to, someone who's been through it themselves. Hooking your parent up with a support group can make a terrific difference to their ability to cope, and their happiness and peace of mind (see guides in Chapters 2 and 3). Whether or not your parents have outside help, the responsibility is horrendous, especially for someone who may be quite frail themselves.

If your parents are in this situation try to give them a break – have them to stay with you or other members of the family for short periods, or arrange some respite care for a few days. There are charities that provide this, and even organize holidays for carers (see guides at the end of Chapter 3). And remember that carers are entitled to an assessment too (see guides at the end of Chapter 3).

When You Have to Get Involved

Dementia is a nightmare for families. Whether or not you're involved on a daily basis, all the same emotions come into play. Your parents, the strong people who cared for you, now need you to help care for them, and this role reversal is hard to accept. It goes against the grain to step into their lives and interfere.

Stanley's parents, Geraldine and Barry, are still living at home together. They're in their early eighties. His mother has lost a lot of her short-term memory and his father is becoming increasingly frail.

'They both get attendance allowance but they won't use it to pay for help. Dad tries to keep on top of everything. The garden's become a jungle – he manages to cut the grass and gets completely shattered. I visit them three or four times a week but he resents my help. In fact I don't think he even realizes the amount of running about I'm doing to keep them going.

'We buy them ready-meals because they can't cook reliably any more. We had to take the microwave away – it was a disaster. Mum kept putting metal dishes in it. And she set fire to the cooker when she put the deep-fat fryer on the hob and switched on a ring underneath it. It's a good job Dad was there to put it out.

'Mum wanders off when they go to the supermarket. The daily risks are frightening. She's got Crohn's disease which makes her incontinent, but because she can't remember things she doesn't change herself often enough. She used to have an alarm clock set up to go off every hour to remind her, until she couldn't remember what the bell was for.

'I get depressed because they can't maintain their standards. It hurts to see the mess. I go through their fridge and throw away all kinds of things. Mum was a medical secretary and always in control. The person she used to be would be horrified at the state her bathroom is in.'

'Even with all this they apparently don't qualify for regular personal care, although the community nurse comes in every three weeks or so for a chat.

'I'm trying to do it all, hold it together, but the biggest problem is that I have no brothers or sisters, there's only me. My partner Joy is fantastic. She's stronger than I am and says I need to sit down with Dad and talk to him about getting them some help. I'd gladly pay for it – I know they won't. But Dad just keeps on saying he doesn't *need* help.

'I can deal with the extra work; it's the emotional part that's so difficult. You feel you're intruding, but you have no choice because they couldn't manage if you didn't. And you've got to be careful what you take away from them. If you don't leave them some responsibilities, what's the point of life?

'I worry about the future – if something happens to Dad, Mum won't cope, and she's adamant she won't go into a

home. I suppose I'd have to sell her house and mine and move her in with us. But what happens then? I couldn't leave her on her own all day, but I have to go out to work. You find yourself trying to work out which one you'd prefer to die first . . .'

Stanley is finding it hard to come to terms with all this, but it helps that he's aware how important it is to give someone with dementia things to think about and do. He doesn't try to take over, so although his father is offended by his offers of help, they've stayed good friends. It doesn't always happen like that. Sometimes the fear of what's happening to them, plus anger at themselves for being unable to do things, can make your parents lash out at the very people they need most.

Hannah, who was 92, lived just a few doors away from her daughter and son-in-law Alison and Lloyd. She developed Alzheimer's disease and went downhill in a matter of months, becoming aggressive and irrational.

'It caused us no end of frustration. At one moment Mum would get angry because we wanted to help, and the next she'd be hurling abuse at us for never coming to see her – in fact we visited her every day.

'And she'd behave so badly. When we took her shopping for shoes she had a tantrum exactly like a petulant child, sulking, refusing to try them on – "I don't know why I need new shoes".

'She got steadily worse until once in the middle of the night we found her on the floor wedged between the bed and the dressing table. Her coat and walking stick were across the bed – she'd been trying to get up to go to bingo.

'One of the hardest things was to see the stains on her sweater and the crumbs on the floor – she'd always been so house-proud.'

'Mum had lots of wonderful friends, but she'd tell us that they'd abandoned her. To hear her talk you would think she had no friends. We put a diary in her hall and asked everyone to sign it when they'd been so we could show her what was really happening. It was full of names.

'Mum berated us, but in her lucid moments I think she was glad we were close to her. It upsets you but you realize you have no right to be upset. What was going on in her head was beyond her understanding. We tried to get inside her mind – but it wasn't her mind any longer.'

Hannah wasn't angry with Alison and Lloyd, she was angry with herself, and ashamed of the indignity of needing her food cutting up, of things like her teeth not fitting properly as she lost weight, and that she couldn't take care of herself any longer.

After all, how do you come to terms with something like this? You have a lifetime of being in charge of yourself, and suddenly you're like a baby, needing help with the simplest things. You've lost your independence. No wonder you shout at people – your whole world has turned upside down. Alison and Lloyd understood this and were marvellously patient with Hannah, but that patience can be hard to maintain.

When your partner's parent develops dementia, it can put a terrific strain on your relationship. 87-year-old Millicent had Alzheimer's disease, and it drove a wedge between her son Jimmy and his wife Diana.

'We started getting phone calls from the police. Mum would be wandering down the street in her nightie at two a.m. Or the neighbours would phone to say she'd locked herself out, or that she was standing in a local shop, completely lost.

'We'd turn out and rescue her. She never knew what had happened and sometimes she'd yell at us for no reason – a

bit like a rowdy drunk really – fighting mad. In between she seemed normal and could never remember anything about it, but it began to happen more and more often.'

'I talked to her GP and social services, who organized some help for her – getting her meals and checking a couple of times a day that she was all right – while we all talked about whether she needed to go into a home. She wouldn't hear of it, so social services' hands were tied.

'I tried to call in on my way home from work sometimes just to check on her, and Diana would pop in every day – but it meant her dashing out of work at lunchtime, and sometimes Mum would be rotten to her when she got there, accusing her of plotting and interfering and saying she didn't need the help. But of course she did – she'd let pans boil dry, and often messed herself.

'My wife got fed up because it was always us who had to deal with Mum – we're only round the corner and my sister lives miles away.

'I tried to get my sister to do more but she wouldn't have it and in the end we had a row. I'm afraid I didn't always keep my temper with Mum either, because Diana was doing so much and the responsibility was wearing her down – as she said, it wasn't even her own mother.

'It all built up until Diana and I started to fight. She accused me of taking advantage of her. I hadn't meant to, but Mum was ill – what could I do? In the end she said she couldn't stand it any longer and left me. Mum's dead now, but I'm still not speaking to my sister – I think if she'd done her share with Mum I might still be married.'

Maybe there were other things going on in Diana and Jimmy's marriage, but Millicent's dementia was enough to tip the scales into disaster. Jimmy blames himself as much as his sister for his divorce and asks himself how it could have been different, but the fact is he was reacting to circumstances – there's no way to plan neatly. It's vital to keep talking to each other instead of fighting about it. And while it's true that Jimmy's sister lived too far away to be called out at night, she could have helped at weekends, and maybe a couple of evenings a week.

If you find yourself in this situation with your family, have a conference and ask everyone to do their bit. There might well be some reluctance – it's not a pleasant job – but you'll get further if you keep your temper and make reasonable requests based on people's circumstances. Getting cross and making demands will just give them an excuse to refuse.

Going into hospital can be particularly frightening and traumatic for someone with dementia, especially if they can't communicate very well. Hospital is worrying enough for any elderly person (see Chapter 5) but the combination of being unwell, plus the disorientation of being in a strange place among strange people and the disruption of their routine, might make dementia symptoms worse.

Have a chat with the hospital social worker, or the nurse who will be in charge of your parent's case and explain what their symptoms and behaviour usually are, what they like/dislike to eat and so on. In theory these should all be covered by your parent's GP, but in practice it's better to make sure everyone knows everything.

When You Have to Do the Coping

Having a parent with dementia to live with you will put you all under a lot of pressure. It will affect every single area of your life and that of your partner and your children, so it's something to think about seriously before you take it on, even temporarily.

Arnold was in the early stages of dementia when his wife Eve went into hospital. His son Ian and daughter-in-law Nicole had Arnold to stay with them until she came out.

Nicole says:

'It seemed the obvious thing to do. Ian's mum was going to be out of action for a few months and we knew Arnold would have trouble managing on his own. We didn't want him to have to go into a home short term.

'Arnold was a smashing man. I'd known him for decades and loved him dearly, but having him around all the time was much harder than I thought it would be. It wasn't that he tried to be difficult – he was marvellous – always good-tempered and appreciative.

'He was very forgetful, but not completely incapable, and could dress himself and take a shower. He even went for walks, although he'd get down the drive and stand, sometimes for several minutes, trying to remember whether to go left or right. I'd watch him from the window, dying to go out and help him, but knowing that he had to do it for himself. It was heartbreaking.

'He'd want to help with chores. I'd walk into the kitchen to find him trying to wash up or make a cup of tea, but he couldn't see very well and his co-ordination was poor. I dreaded him cutting or scalding himself. If I had to go out I'd worry – he could easily have burned the place down. It was like having a toddler in the house – he was never off my mind and I hardly dared let him out of my sight.

'Arnold wasn't unhappy – in fact he seemed quite content, and on his good days we'd often have a laugh together. But those flashes of his old self just made it harder.

'Little things got under my skin. I'd want to snap at him, and although I never actually did snap, I'd feel so *guilty*. I'd ask myself, what sort of a person are you? You know it's not his fault. I'm ashamed of it, but I can't deny that the irritation was there. I'd find myself giving him little lessons on how to do things but of course they never made any impression. I just wanted him to be his old independent self – and he couldn't be.

'It was hard on Ian too but he was at work, and sometimes away on business for a few days at a time so I'd be completely alone with Arnold. I wondered how on earth Eve found the strength to cope, day in, day out. Loving her husband could only make it tougher, not easier.

'Sometimes I'd get up in the mornings feeling panicky, dreading the day ahead. It was the emptiness that was so difficult to watch. Arnold would sit for hours, just dozing or staring into space. Being in close contact with a mind that's falling apart, watching someone you care about cease to exist as a person, is like being in a twilight zone – it's unreal.

'I'm glad we were able to look after Arnold, and I'd do the same again, but I know now absolutely I couldn't have taken him permanently – it would have felt like a life sentence.'

Nicole shouldn't blame herself for her feelings. The closer you are to someone, the harder it is to watch. And the helplessness of being unable to do anything about it makes you angry. Try to remember that it's fate you're angry with, not the person themselves.

Tracy and Jason had her widowed father Sonny to live with them when his dementia became severe.

'It never occurred to us not to have him. I thought, he's my dad – I can't put him in a home. He stayed with us until he died, he was happy and I'm so glad we did it, but I had no idea what it would be like. I was frantic with worry about him all the time, and the physical side of it was awful. He became incontinent, and although his care worker would change his pads, it was a woman and Dad hated that; he couldn't bear the idea of her getting so personal. It would upset him so much.'

It's true that most care workers are women, which many elderly men find difficult to deal with, but don't let that prevent you from taking the help that's available, even if it means you have to be selective about the jobs they do.

When it comes to making a decision about whether or not to look after a parent with dementia, sometimes instinct kicks in. Pauline's father died and her mother Chrissie became too mentally frail to take care of herself.

'When we realized Mum would need looking after I made enquiries about nursing homes straight away. I have a sister but I knew the only person who would take Mum would be me, and I didn't want to do it.

'She didn't really want to go into a home but I persuaded her. It wasn't that I didn't care, but I know I'd have nagged her. On top of that my job involves fantastically long hours and horrendous deadlines, and I can't afford not to work. Mum needed someone there all the time so I felt I had to get her into a home. But if I'm honest I know I was rationalizing the decision to myself and I feel terribly guilty about it now she's dead.

'I keep telling myself that if I'd tried I could have found a way to do at least some of my job from home, but it all seemed too complicated at the time. Half of me felt I should have her, the other half was telling me not to. But I promised Dad I'd look after Mum and I didn't. I should have had her with me.'

The panic Pauline felt at the prospect of having her mother to live with her was based on real self-knowledge. She could imagine herself putting Chrissie under pressure to 'try harder' and she knew this would make them both unhappy. Avoiding this scenario in Pauline's case was common sense.

Sometimes you have to be strong enough to take what can look like a hard decision. It doesn't matter what the world thinks – or even more important, what *you* feel you *should* think. What matters is coming to a solution that will be best for your parents and that you can all live with.

The sheer amount of work involved in caring for someone with dementia is hard to imagine. If you're permanently exhausted and stressed out, if your nights are interrupted, if you have no one to share your anxieties with, your life can become almost unbearable.

Cath's grandfather Vincent was diagnosed with Alzheimer's disease when he was 80. Her mother Roseanne lived near him, and took care of him for ten years.

'Granddad became a grumpy old man and wasn't easy to deal with. He'd imagine people were going behind his back. He'd ring Mum in the middle of the night. She could never go on holiday because she daren't leave him.

'When it was clear he couldn't live at home any more Mum tried to find a care home for him, but his dementia was very severe and it took her months.

'The home isn't very good. One day we found Granddad lying on a mattress on the floor just quivering, with a dirty continence pad. Mum feels guilty, and asks herself whether she'd have sent him there if she hadn't been desperate. Granddad is too frail to move anywhere else now, and anyway, where would she send him?

'After watching Mum go through all this I don't want my children to do the same thing for me. I say, take a long-term view. Before I get to that stage put me in a care home I'm happy with, and don't worry too much about whether they'll keep me if I lose my mind completely – it won't bother me much by then, will it?'

Cath's attitude has been brought about by seeing at close quarters what her mother has suffered, and by worrying about her grandfather, but you don't have to put up with neglect like this.

If you're not satisfied with the care home your parent is in, take it up with the manager. Homes are inspected twice a year by the Care Standards Authorities (see guides in Chapter 4) and any criticisms have to be taken seriously, so if you're still not happy, contact them direct.

It's true there's a shortage of care homes that will take severe dementia patients, and that some areas are much better served than others. Check prospective homes carefully (see guides in Chapter 4). People with dementia are especially vulnerable because they can't speak up for themselves. A good home, on the other hand, will have staff who truly understand what your parent is going through, and know how to provide an environment in which they can be happy and free from anxiety.

If your parents are in a home there are things you can do to make their lives happy. Irene is 85 and widowed. Since she's been in her care home she's had several strokes and has gradually lost most of her short-term memory and some of her ability to communicate with people. Her children and their families all make long trips to visit her, including her granddaughter, Saffron.

'Grandma comes and goes. Sometimes you can visit her and she's lively and chatty, although she'll be talking normally and then suddenly veer off into nonsense. Then at other times she can hardly talk at all and just lets everything wash over her. You never know what she's going to be like, but she does always seem to know who we are.

'She never remembers who's been to see her but that doesn't put us off. After all, she's lost her past, she has no

real future – her pleasures can only be in the present, so we try to give her as many happy moments as possible.'

'Everyone visits separately so she gets more bites of the cherry. My brother and I take our kids, who are all under eight. We both have babies, and she lights up when she sees them. When she's well enough she holds them for a minute or two.

'My two eldest girls remember her as she was before she got like this and they're very kind and loving. We've explained to them that Grandma is old and can't talk very well and they're wonderful with her. Her great-grandchildren will remember her after she's gone and I know she'd love that.'

It can be harder for teenagers to accept what's happening to their grandparents or great-grandparents. They're likely to be embarrassed in ways that very young children aren't, and stay away because they don't know what to say or how to behave. They'll also have formed a much longer, stronger relationship with their grandparents, and might find the whole idea too hard to face.

If that's the case with your children, explain how much happiness they'll be giving if they visit; remind them how much their grandparents have always loved them and say how pleased they'd be to see them. You can point out that they don't have to worry about making conversation, just chat about what they've been doing at school, university, football, wherever. Sometimes a hug will be all that's needed to make their grandparents' day.

Gillian's father Lewis was 84 when he went into a home. He had advanced Alzheimer's disease and didn't always recognize her.

'Dad didn't know who I was a lot of the time so I didn't think I was doing him much good, and though I'd planned to go every day, I found myself going two or three times a week instead. It depressed me to see him in that state, made me face how changed he was, and if I'd gone more often I wouldn't have been able to cope. On top of this he'd criticize me to the nurses: "*She's* the one who put me here." It made me cross so I'd make an excuse and leave early rather than show it.

'It was hard too because when he knew me on his good days he'd say, "Please take me home with you – you know I'll be good. Why are you doing this to me?" His mind was in a fog.'

Gillian might have been reluctant to go as often as she'd intended but she still went to see her father a lot. Her feelings illustrate just how easy it is to find reasons to beat yourself up. Do what you can and feel good about it, instead of trying for the impossible and failing. Then you'll be less likely to duck out altogether.

In some families the fact that their parents don't always remember they've been to see them, or accuse them of imagined neglect, can cause resentment, even jealousy – why have they remembered her visit and not mine? Why have they been telling everyone I never come to see them?

If you're tempted to feel resentful, remember, dementia has deprived your parent of the ability to join thoughts together. They don't love you less – but they do need you more.

The practical complications of dealing with a parent who has dementia can be daunting. Every case is different and getting help can sometimes be an uphill struggle. The guides overleaf and in Chapters 2 and 3 apply equally to people with dementia, as do Guides 3 to 8 in Chapter 4.

Guide 1 – Facts about Dementia

Organization	What it does
Alzheimer's Society Helpline: 0845 3000336 www.alzheimers.org.uk N. Ireland: 02890 664100 Alzheimer's Scotland Dementia Helpline: 0808 808300 www.alzscot.org	Provides fact sheets on every aspect of dementia.
Alzheimer's Research Trust 01223 843899 www.alzheimers-research.co.uk	Dementia charity. Provides fact sheets and online information
BUPA www.bupa.co.uk	Provides fact sheets on medical aspects of dementia
Stroke Association England/Wales Helpline: 0845 3033100 www.stroke.org.uk N. Ireland: 0845 7697299 Chest, Heart and Stroke Scotland: 0845 0776000	Provides information and fact sheets on strokes and dementia caused by strokes
MIND (National Association for Mental Health) Information line: 0845 7660163 www.mind.org.uk N. Ireland Association of Mental Health: 02890 328474 www.niamh.co.uk Scottish Association of Mental Health: 0141 5687000 www.samh.org.uk	Provides fact sheets
Health Promotion England: www.hpe.org.uk Health Promotion Division, National Assembly for Wales: 02920 752222 www.hpw.wales.gov.uk Health Education Board for Scotland: 0131 5365500 www.hebs.scot.nhs.uk	Provides reports, leaflets, booklets on various aspects of dementia

Guide 2 – Where to Get More Information

Organization	What it does
Social Services (see local phone book)	Organises assessment to determine level of care needed Provides assessment for carers
NHS for NHS continuing care	Talk to your GP about assessment
Benefits Agency Social Security (see local phone book) Benefit Enquiry Line: 0800 882200	Will help you find out if you are entitled to extra benefits and exemption from council tax
Continence Foundation www.continencefoundation.org.uk	Provides information and fact sheets
Incontact (continence advice) 0870 7703246 www.incontact.org email: info@incontact.org	Provides information and support
Office of the Public Guardian www.guardianship.gov.uk England/Wales: 0845 3302900 Scotland: 01324 678300 N. Ireland: Office of Care and Protection: 02890 724733	Provides information on the law
Carers UK For booklets: 020 7490 8818 CarersLine: 0808 8087777 www.carers.org	Provides support and information for carers Booklets Helpline

At a Glance

- Get an early diagnosis
- Arrange for an assessment – and one for the carer if necessary
- Try not to take over – leave them some responsibilities
- Keep them stimulated
- Don't tell them to try harder
- Respect their dignity
- Keep your temper – be patient
- Remember they can't help their lapses
- They might qualify for continuing NHS care

Chapter 7

THINKING ABOUT THE FUTURE

Families are remarkable. Whether they're surrounding us with love or causing us untold anguish, they're at the root of our existence. We might be scrapping with them like prizefighters; we might have refused to speak to them for years; they could be scattered so widely we hardly know them. Or we might be close friends, sharing wonderful family gatherings, talking incessantly about things we have in common. Whether it's one of these extremes or somewhere in the middle, the plain fact is that family dynamics matter to us. Our relationship, or lack of one, with our relatives affects our lives profoundly; it informs our choices and augments or diminishes our overall happiness.

In modern families, with all their fragmentation, extension and complexity, it can often be the existence of our parents that keeps the glue in the joints. They're conduits for information, a reason to meet; they can shame us into belonging. Once they start to move off centre stage the family unit can simply fall apart.

And unfortunately, coinciding with this potential meltdown, various legal issues raise their ugly heads. There's nothing, absolutely nothing, like a will for dividing families into factions. Then there's the question of power of attorney – that's a goody for producing sibling rivalry. Add to this heady cocktail the question of what, if anything, your parents want to do about end-of-life decisions like withdrawal of treatment, and you've got a mixture that can be fatal to family relations.

It isn't necessarily a matter of who gets the money, the house, the Staffordshire pot dogs; it's about facing the reality that our parents *will* die and dealing with that in emotional terms, as well as practical. It's about wanting what's best for our parents, and not always agreeing about what the best is – with them, and/or with everyone else.

But family ties are enormously durable. You can break off communication for decades and find it's still possible to come back from that. You can hate each other passionately, be jealous, hold grudges, have blazing rows whenever you're in the same room – but blood *is* thicker than water. Whatever chemical/mystical cord it is that binds families together, it makes a good solid job of it.

Remember that fact if you're tussling with legal matters. They'll only divide the family if you all let them – so don't let them.

Have They Made a Will?

If you make your will earlier in life when death is still something that happens to other people, it doesn't seem like a big deal. You might even revisit it to make alterations as your circumstances or feelings change; you're used to its existence; it's business, a fact of life, not of death.

But if you start thinking about a will when you're old, it's something else altogether. It's a concrete admission of your mortality. Of course your parents might have come to terms with this, made their will and got on with their lives. But for many elderly people a will can have all kinds of uncomfortable – even unthinkable – connotations. It can almost amount to superstition. If I make a will, if I admit to myself in writing that one day I'm going to die, then I *will* die. What was wispy, vague, ignorable, becomes a frightening – and imminent – reality.

'I don't want to think about dying – why would I? I'm going to find out all about it soon enough. My family can sort my stuff out when I'm gone. I'll be past caring then, won't I?' – Myrtle, aged 87

It's tempting to discount an attitude like Myrtle's, to brush it aside and try to jolly your parents along. But what she's feeling isn't just fear but sadness, and maybe just a tiny little bit of resentment that the rest of the world will be alive and she won't. The human mind finds it hard to be totally logical on the subject of death.

There you are, long past middle age – further past it than you like to admit, even to yourself. Everyone around you is encouraging you to 'be sensible' and tidy up the loose ends in your life 'before it's too late' or 'while you still can'. You know they're right, but the prospect of actually doing it feels unpleasant. You're reluctant because you're being forced to contemplate a world without you in it, the people you love going on and you not being there with them . . . perhaps quite soon.

It's a sad fact that wills can lead to strife when what they're actually meant to do is prevent it. And the strife sometimes happens before the person who's made the will has actually died – or even before the will has been made in the first place.

That doesn't alter the fact that it's better to have a will than to die intestate – for all kinds of reasons, emotional as well as practical. It enables your parent, rather than the state, to make the decisions about who gets what, and this can be important if they're not married to their partner or they want to leave something to a friend. It can matter from a tax point of view, too.

It's worth checking out the laws of inheritance where your parents live because England and Wales differ in some respects from Scotland, and Northern Ireland could be different again.

If you bring up the subject of wills and your parents won't have it, you need to find a different strategy (see Chapter 1). If you just keep harping on about it you risk them telling you to stop nagging, then you start to get irritated – cue family row.

Sandy's father Clifford was 87 and refused to take any action at all.

'Dad wouldn't even discuss making a will. It worried me because he's been married twice and there are stepchildren and half-brothers all over the place, but he just kept saying no and getting mad with me.

'In the end we fell out. I told him he could stew in his own juice – I was only trying to help. We all have short tempers in our family and I knew that sorting out Dad's estate would be a nightmare when he died. I wasn't wrong. No one was satisfied – everybody felt Dad had short-changed them. It upset me because I don't like to think of him being remembered that way. He was a generous man.'

If Clifford had realized this would happen he might have been prepared to reconsider. It's natural to want your family to remember you with affection. But with so many different relationships to think about, so many people's feelings to take into account, he might well have been shying away from all the decisions as just too difficult and exhausting.

Sandy could have tackled this by explaining in a low-key way that he was worried the family might fall out if Clifford didn't make a will. And he could have offered to organize a meeting for his father with a solicitor, making a point of saying he'd keep out of things himself if that was what his father wanted.

Unfortunately Sandy took a stand. He felt he was in the right so he never made it up properly with his father – something he regrets now.

'When I look back it was only a will – what did it matter? It wasn't worth fighting over, and I lost my dad for good.'

In fact what Sandy and Clifford were battling about was control – Clifford thought Sandy was trying to take over, and Sandy thought he knew best. A quiet chat would have been far more effective than a forceful argument. A measured discussion would have implied both sides were equal.

Clem and Berenice are in their eighties and they've made a formal will precisely because they wanted the pleasure of deciding who gets what.

'We'd already made out one of those will forms but it didn't feel secure somehow. There are so many people in the family and we'd like to remember them separately so we felt we really ought to have a proper will. There isn't much to leave, but we like to think that our family will get the things we want them to have and that *they'd* want to have.

'And you know, the solicitor was so helpful and made it all so simple. She chatted to us about what we wanted to do and then explained everything. We feel better now it's all taken care of.'

If your parents are receptive to the idea of a will – even if they're not so keen – once you've broached the subject it's worth giving them some literature. There's plenty of information available spelling out the advantages in an impartial manner that's difficult to ignore. You can chat it over with them when they've read it, but the impetus will be coming from them not you, so they'll still be in control.

It's important they feel they're in charge. Your parents have always dealt with their own affairs. They won't want to change that. It could be hard for them to ask for – and accept – input from someone they've always seen as needing *their* guidance.

But they could be in need of a sounding board. It might not be easy to decide who gets what. If you were in your parents' place you'd probably want to talk to someone about it. How would you choose which member of the family to discuss it with? If they don't get on with each other, or you don't get on with some of them, you might be afraid the rows you were hoping to avoid by making a will would start as soon as you singled out one member of the family to confide in.

Guy's mother Fanny had never mentioned the subject.

'Mum was 85 and I hadn't a clue what she'd done about a will, if anything. We hadn't always been the closest of friends and I was a bit wary of bringing it up in case she thought I was being pushy. Then she broke her hip and, I don't know, it suddenly hit me that she was old.

'I told my sister Toni that I was worried and she laughed and said Mum had made a will when she was 80, making her the executor. I should have been glad, but I was hurt. Why hadn't Mum chosen me? Why hadn't my sister told me?'

Guy felt excluded by his mother but from her point of view it was natural to talk to the daughter she felt close to rather than the son who often bickered with her and who might have started to argue. Fanny wasn't signalling that she didn't love Guy – just that she felt more comfortable confiding in her daughter. It might have helped if Toni had mentioned the will to her brother – but Fanny had specifically told her not to do so in case Guy got angry.

You can't really blame your parents if they're reluctant to tell you what they have to leave. You wouldn't be so keen to give them your financial details, would you? It's more than just private – it's intimate. People draw conclusions and make all kinds of judgements about you based on your financial situation. It may be regrettable, but it's human nature. The instinct to keep it to yourself can sometimes be dead right.

Being forced to think of your parents in terms of what they own changes your perception of them, and of yourself. It subtly alters your relationship with them, in your mind and in theirs.

They might be feeling insecure, wondering why you want to get involved. 'Are they more bothered about the money than me? Don't they love me? Won't they miss me when I'm gone?'

You could get the family together and suggest you all go to your parents and explain, en masse, why they don't have to worry; that whatever decisions they take are all right with you; that it's their money to do what they like with.

Barnaby and Poppy, who are almost 90, have told their daughter Daphne that they've sorted everything out.

'Mum and Dad are very proud of the fact that they've made a will and they've given us all the details of what's in it. They've been saving for years – not for their old age, but so they can pass it on to *us*. They live very plainly and won't take nice holidays, even though they could afford them.

'My sons and I have told them just to get on and spend it on themselves, not to worry about us – but they don't *want* to spend it. They just keep saying it's a nice little nest egg for our future.

'We tell them that we want them to live as long as possible to have time to spend every penny – after all, they've earned that right.'

For Poppy and Barnaby, being able to pass on something to their family is a matter of pride. They're not showing off; they see it as their role. 'We're your parents and it's our job to look after you – we want you to be safe when we're gone.'

If your parents are in this frame of mind, it can help to get all the family into one room with them and tell your parents you want them to stop worrying about you. But be careful not to make them think what they have to leave is insignificant or unimportant to you. Don't say 'we don't want/need your money'. Explain instead that it will make you all very happy to look back and think they had everything they could possibly want – every comfort, every pleasure. Tell them if they don't it will make you feel you've failed *them*.

Families can work things out. What it needs is some thought for everyone's point of view. Maurice's mother Amy is 95. She's been living with his sister Claire for fifteen years.

'After Dad died Mum sold her house, bought one with my sister and made a fresh start. They live a few hours' drive away from me so, although I see them sometimes, Claire takes all the strain. Because of that we agreed that I wouldn't be left anything in her will, that Claire would have it all for looking after Mum for all these years. It's only fair.'

Maurice's unselfish arrangement with his mother will have done a lot to put her mind at rest – she knows everyone's comfortable with what's going to happen.

Of course this might not always be the case. Wills can bring out the worst in people. They're used to settle scores, wreak revenge and show spite.

Wills sometimes bring out jealousy and cause deep rifts in the family – 'Why did Mum leave that to my sister? She always promised it to *me*.' But what you're feeling here isn't so much envy or greed as insecurity and rejection – 'Didn't Mum love me as much as my sister?' In fact, the chances are your mother might simply have forgotten a promise made years before – or thought she was being fair. Don't look for slights too hard and you won't find them.

Gordon was so sure his family would fight over his possessions he took unusual steps to prevent it. His great-nephew Jay remembers it with a smile.

'Great-uncle Gordon had no children. He made my dad his executor and told him that he'd mortgaged the house and it would revert to the mortgage company when he died. He said that his will was going to allow everyone to choose two things each from the house contents – but they'd have to pay market price for them. As executor my dad had to keep this a secret from the rest of the family, dreading the row that he was pretty sure would ensue.

'After Uncle Gordon died the local auctioneer came in and valued the contents and the family all bought two items each. Everything left over was sold off too and the money divided between them.'

Whether or not Gordon's family *would* have fought if he'd left a more usual will is a moot point. The irony is they fell out anyway because they were suspicious that Jay's father had somehow got more than they had.

'Poor old Dad had to take a lot of flak, which wasn't fair because Uncle Gordon had treated him just like the others.'

Gordon's rather drastic solution wouldn't appeal to everyone – and in fact it didn't keep the peace at all. But although he didn't realize it himself, making a will like that wasn't really about preventing a row; it was about being able to carry on influencing people and events after his death.

Your parents might decide they'd rather do at least some of their giving while they're still alive to enjoy it, although there's a limit to what they can hand over. Honor is 90 and lives in a care home.

'When I sold my flat to move here I knew I'd have to get rid of most of my bits and pieces, so I gave it to my family. My son and daughter, my grandchildren and great-nephews and nieces all got things – clocks, china – I had some lovely china.

'I let them all take what they wanted and the youngsters were thrilled to bits. They're students and they needed lots of bits to start them off, so nothing was wasted, even things like tin openers and bread knives. It was a pleasure to see their faces. And it's nice to think my things are being used and appreciated by people I love.'

This kind of pragmatism is rare, but wonderful. Honor's family are surrounded by things that will always remind them of her. They love and admire her, not so much for her generosity as for her courage, positive attitude and young outlook. That's the best kind of influence to have after your death.

Keeping Control

Other decisions your parents might face can be harder to tackle than a will. They involve acknowledging some harsh possibilities they'll have been ignoring – that there might come a time when they're either so ill or mentally incapable that they can't think and act for themselves; that they won't be mentally independent.

Do your parents want to designate someone who, if this situation should arise, will have the legal right to make decisions for them? They might not much fancy the idea of discussing a scenario such as this, but it's worth having a family conference with them to talk through the subject. As long as you're careful not to push them into anything, then going through the pros and cons and explaining what's available to them under the law can be reassuring rather than threatening. Once again, knowledge is power. They may well decide they don't want to take any steps at all, but the decision will have been theirs.

The law varies across the UK. England and Wales have the Mental Capacity Act 2005, effective from April 2007; Scotland has the Adults with Incapacity (Scotland) Act 2000; Northern Ireland has the Mental Health Order (NI) 1989. While it's fair to say all three are broadly similar, there are differences, particularly in details and procedures.

What they all provide for is the ability for your parents to give someone the power of attorney to make financial decisions on their behalf should they cease to able to do so themselves.

In England and Wales this is called 'lasting power of attorney'. It encompasses financial matters but it can also, if your parents want it and under certain circumstances, specify their wishes concerning aspects of their own health and welfare, including issues like withdrawal of treatment and resuscitation. Effective from April 2007, this lasting power of attorney has superseded the Advance Directive (Living Will), and the old 'enduring power of attorney' (EPA), although existing EPAs are still legal.

In Northern Ireland, enduring power of attorney covers only financial matters. There is no specific legislation for health and welfare matters; they're dealt with under common law as Advance Directives (Living Wills). But the Act is under review, and may eventually end up very similar, if not identical, to the English Act. If your parents live in Northern Ireland you'll need to check where they are with this.

In Scotland, 'continuing power of attorney' covers financial matters, and 'welfare power of attorney' deals with health and welfare issues.

Money matters

Power of attorney to deal with financial matters is relatively straightforward wherever you live in the UK, although there are grey areas so it's a good idea for your parents to consult a solicitor. Giving someone power of attorney is a highly significant step, and one that can have an enormous impact on the whole family.

Lasting power of attorney (and its Scottish and Northern Irish equivalents) allows a person (or people) chosen by your parents to make decisions about their money: their savings, selling their house, paying bills, whatever your parent wants to include. It has to be made when they still have full mental capacity.

If they wish it can be effective immediately, from the moment the document is signed, or they can state that powers are to be withheld until they become incapable of managing for themselves. At that point the lasting power of attorney has to be registered. Precisely where, how and with whom depends on whereabouts in the UK your parents live.

There are good reasons for taking out this kind of power of attorney. It will remove from your parents the fear that their affairs will fall into chaos.

Janine's father Humphrey had advanced Alzheimer's, and it became clear he couldn't act for himself any longer, so she and her husband Freddy registered the enduring power of attorney they'd all had drawn up a few years before.

'Dad couldn't even get to the bank to cash his own cheques, so we were able to take all that strain from him.'

Janine and Freddy didn't need to make any huge financial decisions on Humphrey's behalf, because he lived in his own home until he died.

Emma's mother Kirsten took out an enduring power of attorney when she was 90.

'Mum wanted to alter her will because she'd sold her house, so we went to see her solicitor. He asked her if she'd given me enduring power of attorney and suggested that it might be a good idea.

'Her immediate reaction was no. She said she didn't want to because it would take her freedom away from her and there wouldn't be any point in living if she couldn't make her own decisions.

'The solicitor explained that with an enduring power of attorney she could keep control, but that if there came a time when she wasn't able to act for herself, I would be ready and everything could go smoothly.

'Her sight is so bad now she can't sign documents, so we've registered the power of attorney, and I've taken over. She still isn't awfully keen because she likes to be independent, but she agreed because she knew it made sense.'

Emily and Hugh's parents, Gavin and Harriet, are in their late eighties, and Gavin resisted the idea to begin with.

Emily says:

'Mum was fine but Dad had been suffering for a while from Alzheimer's. We talked to them about us taking out an enduring power of attorney as it was then, so that if he got worse we could handle things for him and it wouldn't all be dumped on Mum.

'Mum thought it was a good idea but Dad wouldn't consider it. He said he didn't need any interference, he could manage his own affairs. We left it alone, but then Mum told him she wasn't well enough any longer to cope with financial decisions if anything happened to him, and persuaded him to change his mind. He agreed and we took out separate EPAs for both of them.

'Dad's Alzheimer's got worse quite quickly and then Mum went into hospital. While she was there she kept having panic attacks and insisting that Dad sell the house. Eventually he actually went to see an estate agent and told them to put the house on the market.

'Fortunately we'd registered Dad's EPA by then, and so we were able to tell the agent not to do it. Dad was still living there and Mum was going to be coming home! If we hadn't been legally able to act, their house might have been sold round them.

'In fact, Mum became very frail and they went into a care home together. We had to sell the house at that point to pay their fees. Dad died not long afterwards and Mum has dementia now too, so it's fortunate we broached the subject when we did.'

Hugh and Emily both became attorneys, which is what their parents wanted. They're a close family and it felt right for them to have the responsibility jointly. They haven't disagreed about decisions, and they work together in their parents' best interests.

It's not always so easy for anyone to choose the right attorney. You need to have enormous trust in that person and their ability to run your finances when you're in no position to interfere. Even if you're a close family this can cause jealousy between siblings.

Nellie's children, Liza and Kenneth, were both happy she agreed to take out an LPA, but each thought *they* should be her attorney. Liza was upset when Nellie picked her brother.

'I'm the elder child and I thought I should be her attorney, but Mum said that since Kenneth runs his own business it made sense for him to do it because he has more financial experience. I was upset – I'm just as intelligent as my brother and after all, it's not exactly rocket science is it, selling the house and things like that?

'I felt passed over, as though somehow I wasn't good enough to handle it. Kenneth said, rather smugly, that it isn't important who does it, and I tell myself he's right, but it still hurts.'

It would have been more tactful if Nellie had chosen both her children to act for her, either in everything, or dividing up the responsibility. Or she could have got round the problem by selecting someone from outside the family altogether – a friend or a solicitor.

In any case, having more than one attorney can be a safe-guard against bad – or greedy and selfish – decisions. Your parents can decide just how much power they give to their attorneys. Explain all this to them but remember they have to feel completely comfortable about their choice.

Pierre and Jacqueline found choosing their attorneys easy. They're in their early eighties.

Pierre says:

'For a long time we'd been reluctant to think about the sub-ject, and only started to address it seriously quite recently. We gave the job to my son and his wife. They live nearest to us. My daughter lives in France with her family and although she cares about us, she's just not here to do things.'

This kind of solution works well, but your parents might nat-urally prefer to make each other their attorney. If so, it's a good idea to suggest they choose at least one other, younger person, in case their partner dies before them.

Welfare and wellbeing

Wherever your parents live in the UK, and whatever Act they come under, the law regarding end-of-life decisions is, frankly, a minefield. Your parents can give written directives or oral instructions, but to whom and under what circumstances needs to be carefully investigated beforehand – their wishes have to be explicit and most people aren't medical experts. What's more, medical techniques advance all the time.

And what the doctors think comes into it too; they have a duty of care to their patients and there's a foggy area involving withdrawal of medicines and refusal of treatments. On top of all this there's the issue of euthanasia (illegal) and assisted suicide (also illegal). However, there are cases of people travelling abroad to countries where the latter is within the law.

In the broadest terms – and you need to check out the details in your parents' part of the UK – you can't use any kind of advance directive to refuse basic nursing care (things like keeping you clean and comfortable); you can't refuse painkillers or food and drink; you can't demand a particular treatment. But in theory you do have a right (although it may not always be legally binding) to say in advance what treatments you *don't* want administered, even if withholding them could mean you die.

You might think you know already what level of existence would be intolerable to you, but you could change your mind. That's why any instructions need to be frequently revisited and kept right up to date. You can think one thing when you're well and quite another when you're ill. It's all fiendishly complex and difficult.

These kinds of questions tend to be raised when advanced dementia or a terminal illness has been diagnosed, or if your parents have religious or cultural beliefs on the subject. It might be tempting just to advise your parents not to go there, but they could have strong views on how they want their life to end.

Prue's mother Irma was only 73 when she had a severe heart attack.

'Mum was very ill. There was extensive damage to her heart and she knew that even if she recovered she'd be in very poor shape physically. But she kept on fighting. There would never have been any question in my mind of non-resuscitation or withdrawal of treatment. I knew very well how she felt. She'd always said, right from when I was young, that if ever it came to that point I was never, never, just to let her die.

'Mum would say to me, "It doesn't matter how ill I am, what state I'm in, even if I can't speak to you, don't ever assume I'd prefer to die or that I'd be better off dead. Life's sweet, and nobody should take it away from you because they think it's best. It won't be best for me."'

'I could never have done anything against those wishes, however hard it might have been for me to watch her suffering. I knew how adamant she was about it.'

If your parents do want to put something in writing or give you instructions about what they want to happen you need to discuss the whole subject at length with them, together with their doctor. Be patient, whether you agree with them or not. And don't let anyone bully them – in whatever direction.

Theresa's aunt, Primrose, was 89 and in hospital after a series of major strokes.

'My aunt was feeling very sorry for herself and she kept

on and on saying, "Just let me die, my life's not worth living any longer." Her doctor decided to teach her a lesson. The next time she brought it up he said, "OK, when would you like? Pick a day." She panicked – she was hysterical. The doctor had to talk her down, and it took a long time to reassure her.

'The doctor had always known my aunt didn't really mean it, and in any case what she was asking for was illegal, but I think he was way out of order to frighten her like that. I wouldn't have allowed him to do it if it had been my mum.'

Theresa is right to resent the upset her aunt was caused. If the doctor had had the sensitivity to talk with Primrose calmly she'd have been able to look at the subject from all sides and realize the impossibility of what she was asking. Instead of being treated like a recalcitrant child, Primrose would have kept her dignity.

Doctors in general wouldn't behave like this. They take the responsibilities involved very seriously indeed, and should be prepared to talk through the ramifications. It's difficult in any case for them to make decisions on things like resuscitation.

Lynne's grandmother Grace was a very frail 89 and still living at home.

'Gran had a major heart attack. She hadn't left instructions about non-resuscitation so the doctor did his best to revive her. He managed it, but in the process he broke a couple of her ribs. He couldn't help it – she was so tiny and delicate. Gran went into hospital but developed an infection and died a fortnight later.

'If the doctor had left Gran alone she'd have passed away quietly. Instead she had two weeks of tubes and pain, then she died anyway. She'd have been better off if she'd been allowed to go the first time.'

As the law currently stands, where there are no specific instructions doctors have to make a judgement call, which might or might not take the family's wishes into account. If your parents do have firm ideas, it's perfectly possible they might want something you don't agree with, or that some of the family approve of and others don't.

Kris's father died quickly, and she didn't have to make any decisions on his behalf.

'As far as I understand it the law lets you allow someone to die, but not actively to end their life, not to take it into your own hands. But what's the difference between taking away and not giving? None, that I can see.

'It troubles me that people are being asked to make these decisions in circumstances that are so traumatic – you're effectively out of control. You could act out of character.'

What Kris is feeling might resonate for some people. Others might think the law should allow more freedom of choice. The debate has raged for many years. But in the end, your parents and, if appropriate you, are the ones who have to decide how to handle this issue, whether to pursue an advance directive or not. The law is equivocal; the morals and ethics involved are multi-layered. There can be no 'correct' answer.

It's vital your family doesn't muddy the waters by arguing amongst yourselves about it. If your parents have a view, the only way forward is to listen properly to what they're saying, and then talk about it without falling out either with them or with each other. If it's a difficult concept for you to get *your* mind round, just imagine how hard it is for your parents to contemplate.

The following guides will give you ways to discover what the law says, but when it comes to 'living wills', don't expect cut-and-dried responses – there aren't any.

Guide 1 – Advice on Making a Will

Organization	What it does
Age Concern England 0800 009966 www.ageconcern.org.uk **Age Concern Cymru** 02920 431555 www.accymru.org.uk **Age Concern Scotland** 0845 1259732 www.ageconcernscotland.org.uk **Age Concern Northern Ireland** 02890 325055 www.ageconcernni.org	Provides fact sheets
Citizens' Advice Bureaux (see local phone book) www.adviceguide.org.uk	Local advice and information on website
DirectGov www.direct.gov.uk	UK government public service information
Lesbian and Gay Bereavement Project 020 7407 3550	Produces a will pack

Guide 2 – Advice on Lasting Power of Attorney and Regional Equivalents

Organization	What it does
Public Guardianship Office England/Wales: 0845 3302900 www.guardianship.gov.uk Scotland: 01324 678300 N. Ireland Court Service: Office of Care and Protection 02890 724733	Provides information on the Mental Capacity Act and equivalents
Citizens' Advice Bureaux (see local phone book) www.adviceguide.org.uk	Gives advice on the law and your rights
Age Concern (England, Wales. Northern Ireland, Scotland as Guide 1)	Provides fact sheets
Alzheimer's Society 0845 3000336 www.alzheimers.org.uk www.alzscot.org Northern Ireland 02890 664100	Provides fact sheets and advice line

Guide 3 – Advice on Advance Directives (Living Wills) and Regional Equivalents

Organization	What it does
Alzheimer's Society As Guide 2	Provides fact sheets and advice line
Public Guardianship Office as Guide 4	Gives information on Mental Capacity Act and equivalents
MIND 0845 7660163 www.mind.org.uk N. Ireland Association Of Mental Health 02890 328474 www.niamh.co.uk Scottish Association Of Mental Health 0141 5687000 www.samh.org.uk	Has advice line, information sheets
Age Concern As Guide 1	Provides fact sheets
Voluntary Euthanasia Society 020 7937 7770	Gives information on living wills, forms of words
Citizens' Advice Bureaux (see local phone book) www.adviceguide.org.uk	Gives information on the law, your rights

Guide 4 – Advice on Mental Capacity Law Across the UK

Where	Organization
England and Wales	**Office of Public Guardianship** 0845 3302900 (As Guide 2.) www.dca.gov.uk **Citizens' Advice Bureaux** (see local phone book) www.adviceguide.org.uk **Age Concern** England as Guide 1 Wales as Guide 1
Scotland	**Office of Public Guardianship, Scotland** 01324 6783000 www.publicguardianship-scotland.gov.uk **Mental Welfare Commission** www.mwcscot.org.uk **Age Concern Scotland** as Guide 1 **Citizens' Advice Bureaux** (see local phone book)
Northern Ireland	**Office of Care and Protection** 02890 724733 **The Law Centre** 02890 244401 **Help The Aged Seniorline** 0808 8087575 **Age Concern Northern Ireland** as Guide 1 **Citizens' Advice Bureaux** (see local phone book) **Alzheimer's Society** as Guide 2

At a Glance – Wills

- Discuss the benefits of making a will
- Don't crowd your parents
- Let them know it's their choice
- Don't fight amongst yourselves
- Accept your parents' decisions

At a Glance – Lasting Power of Attorney

- Talk it through with your parents
- Check out the law
- Explain the benefits
- Make sure they understand what it means
- Help them choose attorneys they feel comfortable with

At a Glance – Advance Directives and Equivalent

- Check out the law
- Listen to your parents
- Try to stay calm
- Make sure they understand what they're doing
- Keep checking they haven't changed their mind

Chapter 8

SELLING THEIR HOME

Human beings have a natural nesting instinct. Whether we live in a nomadic tent or a stately home, we embellish our surroundings. If we're nomads we have to restrict ourselves to the portable, but otherwise we can abandon all restraint and decorate to our heart's content.

And we do. We express our personality, indulge our tastes, reveal our inner needs in a way we would never do in any other context, because our home is an extension of ourselves. We aren't just making a style statement – pretty, chic, funky – we're marking our territory; we're saying 'this is *mine*'.

We're very territorial. We'll go to war to protect our home if necessary. It's worth fighting for because it's the one place in the universe where we don't need to pretend. We come through that door and whether we've been trekking the Himalayas or the local high street, we breathe a sigh of relief, put the kettle on and kick back. Home at last!

It's a secret place – it knows us intimately. We make love in it, shout, swear, laugh and cry in it. We stand naked in front of its mirrors and pull in our stomach; sing opera in the shower. We share our thoughts with the wallpaper; lie awake in the dark, worrying. It sees us at our weakest, when we're too ill to get out of bed. It's safe.

Buying a home is an almost universal ambition and we save with dedication to do it. If we manage to achieve it we relax, even though it's the biggest purchase most of us will ever make and can keep us financially chained for decades – perhaps for life. But we think it's worth it.

With so much of ourselves invested – emotionally, spiritually and literally – we're likely to hang onto our home like billyoh. All the more so if someone is trying to talk us out of it and into somewhere we don't want to be; if we're old and chunks of our lives have already started falling away; or if our life partner has died and we're left there all alone. The idea of leaving it is unbearable. We're going to cling to the doorframe with our fingernails, swallow the house key, hide under the bed, do anything to stay in our haven.

But the hard fact remains – one day, maybe soon, your parents could need you to be that someone, winkling them out of their shell and bringing them, vulnerable and afraid, into the open. You won't like doing it, even when you know it's for the best, but you'll find the strength, because you love them.

Broaching the Subject

Unless they've already brought it up themselves, it can be hard to tackle the subject of selling with your parents. If they're becoming too infirm to live alone, selling the house could be just one part of a shattering life change that's going to tear their world apart. Whether what's being contemplated is downscaling to sheltered housing, a move in with you or into a care home, it's going to be an unwelcome prospect and how you tackle the whole subject depends on your parents' situation (see Chapter 4).

Because of the way local authorities finance residential care for the elderly, their home often has to be sold to pay for it (see

Chapter 4), and this means your parents, or you on their behalf, can be hurried into acting. There's no choice, even though none of you will have come to terms with the idea.

That's tough enough, but there are financial things to watch out for too. For example, if one of your parents is in a care home and the other sells their family home, some local authorities might want to count part of the money from the sale in the first parent's means test. As with so much of this, it's not straightforward, so it's worth checking out what happens in your parents' area (see guides at the end of Chapter 4).

Even if they're fit and just need somewhere smaller than the home they're currently rattling around in, they could resent any suggestion they move as an insult. Why is it necessary? What's wrong with keeping things as they are? They've always managed – they're not finished yet. And anyway, it's their *home* – it's *their* home.

As long as your parents continue to live where they lived when they *weren't* old, in their mind they *aren't* old. They can kid themselves nothing has changed. They're the same people, surrounded by the same things – the neighbours, the street. It's their turf.

And it's not an illusion – in many ways things *haven't* actually changed. They might find coping a bit harder, but on the other hand their environment is familiar to them, which can help to compensate for that.

Their daily reality is closely linked at every level to the place they call home. They get up in the morning from the same side of the bed, walk the same route across the kitchen to make a cup of tea and probably take it to the same chair to drink. They're likely to sit in the same place at the table, put the newspaper and TV listings down on the same spot. The chores take a similar shape every day. And why wouldn't they? The house itself hasn't changed. It inflicts its own conventions on its occupants. This doesn't mean your parents are boring creatures with no imagination or initiative, stuck in a mindless rut – far from it. In fact it doesn't just apply to the elderly – we're all creatures of habit to some extent. We fall into patterns that are in themselves reassuring, reaffirming. They give structure to our world, they're comforting, and the busier, the more chaotic and stressful our lives, the more we need those patterns to lean on. We're on autopilot – we're at home.

For your parents, living in a world that has ceased to value their working contribution and is increasingly sidelining them, their home, whether they've lived there for three years or thirty, gives them a purpose – it needs them. They have a responsibility to it, and this means *they're* still important.

Selina's father Des is 78.

'Mum went into a care home with Alzheimer's disease, and Dad has stayed on in the house they shared for fifty years. It's a big place with a large garden but he's managing, with a cleaner and gardener. He helps to run a local business a couple of days a week and plays golf, but his main interest is the garden. He's always been keen; he's out there every day.

'We want him to sell the house and buy something smaller because we're worried he won't have enough energy to keep on doing everything he enjoys. Dad's still comparatively young and if he had somewhere more manageable he should be able to cope for a long time. We suggested it, but he's so attached to the place he wouldn't consider moving.

'Then he came to stay with us for a month and I think it made him realize how lonely he is. We persuaded him to have a look at some properties, but none of them suited him. It's difficult to find a small house with a decent-sized garden.

'There's no point in keeping on about it. We'll leave things for a month or two and then we'll have to try again.'

From Des's point of view, hanging on to the things he enjoys only makes sense. He doesn't want to give up his favourite activity – who would? Selina, on the other hand, is trying to ensure he'll stay fit enough to garden and play golf for many years.

She's right to leave it for a while and try later. The month he spent with her gave him pause for thought and, if Des isn't hassled, he's likely to realize for himself that selling makes sense.

Your parents might resist any idea of a move until illness tips the scales. Donna was struggling to persuade her 80-year-old mother Eleanor to sell her family home.

'When I was growing up my grandparents lived with us. They had the whole of the ground floor. Mum and Grandma were very close – inseparable really – especially after my granddad died. When Grandma herself died in 1969 Mum left everything just as it was – the cupboards were still full of her clothes. Mum wasn't good at moving on.

'Then Dad had a series of strokes which left him incapacitated, and Mum just soldiered on. Looking after him was a terrific strain on her but she didn't tell anyone. I wanted them to move to somewhere easier to manage, but no, they wouldn't think of it. They'd got into these cycles of habit and couldn't seem to break them.

'When Dad died in 2000 Mum was left alone in this house where nothing had changed for decades – some of the furniture was from the 1950s. She was still using paraffin heaters. It was claustrophobic, unhealthy, but she never even thought of selling up and moving.'

'Apart from some arthritis, Mum was a young 74, but she was suffering a lot of stress and never thought of asking for help. She'd just take on too much. And she'd never go near social services. She thought they'd only interfere.

'Then she caught MRSA during a hospital stay and she was very ill. She battled it out but it was a real uphill struggle. I said, "You've got to sell that house – get out of there, start again."

'I finally got her to concede it might be a good idea and we started talking about where she'd like to be. She fancied the seaside but in the end we found somewhere just a couple of miles away from her old house.

'It was hard for Mum to let go but once she did she got this amazing sense of release. She has good neighbours, a little garden – a new life. She's so much happier psychologically that it's like having a new mother. She's a different woman. What I'd say is, even if your parents are resistant, it's worth persevering. The transformation can be amazing.'

Sometimes it can be easier to bury your head and hold on to the past. Eleanor was living her life in retrospect, inside her head. That can be more comforting than moving forward into an unknown future. And the older you get, the more frightening the future can become, because it's shorter – it's got your death in it. Donna knew that moving on was the right thing for her mother so she persisted because she knew that, left to herself, Eleanor would never be able to make the break.

No one would want the decision to be forced by a dramatic downturn in health, so if moving really would be best for your parents, be patient, talk to them about what they'd like if they could wave a magic wand, offer to take them to look at smaller houses; excite them about the prospect of something new rather than daunting them with the differences.

Coming to Terms with It

It isn't just your parents who might have trouble putting the past aside. It can be hard for you to come to terms with the sale of your parents' home.

Daniel is registered blind. He's 90 and has glaucoma. When his wife died he went into a care home and his daughters Bridget and Jilly sold his house.

Bridget says:

'Dad was fine about going into the care home. Mum had looked after him, done his eye drops and everything and he knew that without her he'd never be able to manage. We put his house on the market, but when the sale went through Jilly was upset. I'd never lived there but she had and there were a lot of family memories.'

Part of Jilly's past was tied up in that house. When that's the case you can feel disloyal, that you're turning your back on your own history as well as that of your parents, and this hurts. It can be upsetting too because of what it's saying about your parents – they won't be here forever.

Vera's son Ken wanted his mother to move into a flat near to him.

'Mum had reached 80 without too much trouble but I could see she was struggling. I told her that if she sold the house and came to live near me I'd be able to look in on her most days.

'My brother Tod went berserk. He said it was selfish of me to want to uproot her just to save me the bother of travelling to visit her; that I only wanted her near me so I could work myself into her good books and get the lion's share of her cash – she has quite a lot of money to leave. In fact I'm the one who visits her. I always have been.

'He worked on Mum, saying that she didn't need to sell the house at all, that with a home help she'd be fine. Of course this was what she wanted to hear and she went for it, but it doesn't really work. She's just on the verge of not coping, but my brother's convinced her she's fine. *He's* the one who's being selfish.'

Whether or not Ken's right about Tod being jealous, it's also possible that he just didn't want to see his mother shutting down her life – that it frightened him, and that his instinctive reaction was to persuade her that everything was all right because he *wanted* it to be.

Selling the house is yet another of those situations where families can reach flashpoint. Milly's mother Madge was 79 when she broke her hip and had a lengthy hospital stay.

'Mum really wasn't well when she came out of hospital, so we talked about her selling the house. It wasn't big or fancy but she and her brother had grown up there. She loved it but hadn't been able to keep up with it for a while. She quite liked the idea of a sheltered flat so I put the house on the market while we started looking round for something.

'My Uncle Julian saw the house details in the local paper and went and had a go at Mum. He said the house was "family property" and she had no right to sell it without consulting him. It was rubbish, of course – Mum owned the house outright.

'Mum couldn't stand her ground against him, and I walked into the middle of it. She was in a real state, sobbing her heart out. It made me so furious that I told him a few home truths. I accused him of being jealous, called him a selfish brute and all kinds of horrible things. I dare say I shouldn't have, but he'd upset Mum so much.

'Unfortunately I made things worse. Mum took his side

against me because she said I shouldn't have talked to my uncle like that. I said I was only trying to look after her and then *we* had a row.

'We're friends again now. She's sold the house and she's happy, but she still maintains I was in the wrong about Uncle Julian. Personally, I'll never forgive him.'

It's hard to keep your temper when someone you love is being hurt – your natural instinct can be to wade right in. If Milly had stopped to calm her mother down she'd have been calmer herself when she tackled her uncle and it might have saved rows all round.

Julian certainly had no right to browbeat Madge in that way, but he was probably reacting to the shock of seeing his childhood home on the market. It *was* family property – not legally but emotionally. It didn't occur to Madge but it would have been more considerate to tell him about it beforehand rather than let him find out in that way. The house was hers, but he had some emotional investment in it too.

It isn't easy to decide when is the right time to consider suggesting your parents move. A couple will struggle on together at home but when one of them dies, the other can suddenly find themselves prepared to make a change. Cyril and Martha's daughter Rachael tried to persuade them to sell.

'My parents were very happy in their huge, dilapidated Victorian house. They didn't worry about maintenance – they just let it slowly fall to pieces. The light switches would spark when you turned them on and off.

'Of course it worried us, and we kept hoping they'd see it our way and get rid of the house, but they just wouldn't do it.

'After my father died Mum finally agreed to sell, and we found her a brand-new flat. It was beautifully spacious and light, with a balcony overlooking the town where we lived. But I don't think she ever really came to terms with the move. She used to say, "I'm lonely but I mustn't say that – I know I'm lucky. And I can look down from my balcony and there you all are.'"

Martha's house was demolished after she moved out, and that may have made it harder for her to come to terms with her new life. Everyone has their own way of coping with bereavement – and it *is* bereavement – it's a loss that goes deep. Your home is a part of you, and to lose it and all it contains is to lose a large piece of yourself.

If your parents develop dementia it can be hard to feel sufficiently detached to make decisions.

Christian's father Damien had Alzheimer's disease and it became too severe for him to carry on running his own affairs.

'When Dad was 82 his mind began to deteriorate. He flickered on and off, in and out, so we talked to him and he agreed to let us take up the enduring power of attorney we'd already signed [see Chapter 7]. It was a tough decision for him to make, although he did seem relieved once he'd done it.

'He was looked after at home by wonderful carers, but in his lucid moments he kept saying, "When I get better I'm going to have that boiler seen to" or "I'll have to get the garden straight". It seemed to us that what remained of his sanity was being kept there by the fact that he was in his own home.

'Dad had a stroke and went into hospital. He was very ill for months and the doctors more or less said he wouldn't be coming home, so we sold the house. He didn't know we'd done it and he'd sometimes talk about what he'd do if he did come out. I felt like a criminal, knowing the truth.'

'Dad died in hospital – I don't know if that makes us lucky or not. If he'd recovered enough to come out, I think the shock of the house being gone might have killed him. What does that make me? I don't like to think about it.'

Christian thought he was acting for the best, but it can be difficult to decide what's right under those circumstances. He found all kinds of reasons to justify his decision – the house needed a lot of money spent on it, months of neglect through the winter would have made it worse. But he thinks now it might have been better not to be in such a hurry.

It's possible Christian was simply finding Damien's long illness too much to bear, and needed to take control of *some* aspect of the situation, to feel he was resolving at least something for his father.

If you're faced with a decision like this, think hard, do your best and then don't berate yourself for it. You're only human.

Selling your parents' house can be equally painful *after* they've died. Bella's mother Violet had always said she wanted her family to keep her house on the coast and use it as a holiday home.

'The house was on an island only reachable by ferry, and there was a long and complicated journey for any of us to get to it. We already have a weekend cottage and my brother didn't want one, especially not there, so it was no use to us at all.

'We didn't know how to tell her that. We knew how much she'd have hated the idea, so we let her think we were keeping the house, that we'd all be using it as she wanted. Then after she died we sold it straight away. I conned her really.'

Bella and her family deceived Violet, but they were sure she'd have been completely overthrown by the knowledge that

211

they didn't need or want her house. They did it to spare her, and she died feeling comfortable. Some people might think that's the right thing to do; others that it's better to be honest, that hiding the truth is patronizing. Only you, knowing your parents, can decide which route to take.

If you find yourself faced with a decision like this, try to be honest with yourself. Would you be hiding the truth for your parents' sake, or your own? Of course you'll need to think about what will make them happy *now*, but dig deeper too.

Try to work out what they would have said in their prime about being kept in the dark on important issues. Have they always been the kind of people who faced the truth, however harsh? Or did they prefer to be spared things? Then factor this knowledge into the equation. It might not change your instinctive decision, whatever that is, but you'll have honoured your parents by taking it into consideration.

What about Their Things?

One of the biggest emotional hurdles to selling their house is that your parents won't just be leaving those four walls, but abandoning a whole lifetime's collection of things, and the memories they hold. Imagine how hard that must be.

Think of your own home, all your pieces of furniture and why you like them; your favourite armchair, the piano, the oak chest your grandfather left you, your dining table and chairs, a picture you love – whatever you'd save from a fire. In your head, line up your framed photographs of family and friends. Lots of them, are there? Now select, say, ten things – just ten – to keep, and imagine all the rest going into a black hole for ever . . . hard, isn't it?

Your parents will use various strategies to help them cope with this deprivation.

Ginnie's 83-year-old mother Alma had to be discharged from hospital straight into a care home.

'We hadn't known when she was admitted to hospital that this would be the outcome, and it came as a shock to us all. Mum took it very well. She didn't like the idea, but realized she wasn't well enough to cope alone any longer so she accepted it. It was brave.

'But of course we had to sell her house to pay for her care. She took it on the chin and managed to be stoical about it, but when I offered to take her back there for a few visits to look around and choose what she wanted to keep, she went once and it really upset her. She had a good cry, and then flatly refused to go again.

'She wouldn't talk about why. She just said, "No, you do it." We asked her what she wanted us to bring away but it was hard to get her to tell us even that. To hear her you'd have thought she'd lost interest in everything she owned.

'We made suggestions and gathered up what we thought she'd like, but she didn't seem to be very enthusiastic. She kept saying, "I'm not bothered." When we told her we were giving some of her bigger things to a woman's refuge all she said was, "Good. But don't tell me what you're doing with any of it."'

Alma's way of dealing with a situation she found intolerable was to turn her back on it. If she didn't think about it she wouldn't feel so much pain. To keep on seeing her home and saying goodbye to it would have broken her heart. And to know where her things were going would simply have been too much information – she didn't want to be able to imagine them in their new setting. Her family understood that, and quietly got on and handled it without her.

When Quentin's daughter Marguerite sold his home he reacted quite differently. He was determined to keep everything.

'Dad was adamant that he wouldn't part with anything. It was all going into the care home with him. Of course it wasn't logical or rational – he had a houseful of big old-fashioned furniture. Some of it went right back to when he was young. "They're my memories," he'd say.'

'In the end I was quite ruthless. I got rid of almost all his things. It was hard for Dad, though, saying goodbye to sixty years of his life at once.'

It was difficult for Marguerite too. She had no choice but to take the decisions on his behalf, and he didn't make it easy for her. But what Quentin was really saying was, 'I can't do this – how do I choose between one memory and another? I want them all.'

Marguerite wasn't being ruthless. To have opted out would have been cruel because it would have forced Quentin to make those decisions on his own, to face a future which already felt unbearably bleak.

Sometimes, though, the process can be positive. Natalie's mother Mimi was pleased to get out of her family home and into a flat after her husband died, and Natalie helped her put a new home together.

'We chose, very carefully, my mother's best pieces of furniture and it all looked stunning in her new flat. She was delighted with it. She said that she was learning to appreciate it all over again because in its new setting it looked completely different.'

Doing things this way turned what could have been traumatic into an adventure for Mimi – it was *fun*, and nest building helped to keep her connected to the 'real' active world.

It was lovely for them to be able to share that experience, but it doesn't always work out like that. When Valerie's 80-

year-old mother-in-law Ida developed dementia she went into a care home and her house had to be sold.

'Ida was physically and mentally frail and there wasn't any way she could have sorted out her own things, so we cleared the house for her.

'It felt horrible, walking into that house where I'd always been a visitor, and going through all my mother-in-law's things, while she was still alive and sitting in a chair just three miles down the road. I felt like a burglar and a Peeping Tom rolled into one.'

'Her underwear drawers, airing cupboard, wardrobe – it was all so private, intimate. Have you ever thought about what you keep in the drawer of your bedside table? How personal it is?

'There I was sorting out her kitchen cupboards and pantry, throwing away unopened packets of biscuits, bought when life was normal. I made bundles of the cutlery she'd been polishing for sixty years – and that I'd been dutifully washing up as a visitor for over forty of those. We'd eaten dinner with those knives and forks on the day we told them we were getting married.

'I suppose it might have felt less intrusive if she'd been my mum, but I don't know, even then it would have been uncomfortable. To have to go through Ida's handbags; to find beach bags full of the kind of things you always pack for holidays and then stash away till next time; to unearth press cuttings in the bottom of cupboards, invitations, saved birthday cards – it was as though I had no business there. I learned far more about my in-laws' private life than I felt I had any right to know. Just a few months earlier it would have been unthinkable.

'It seemed as though I was implying she was no longer a person. And then I'd find myself sitting drinking tea with her as if everything were completely ordinary, as if I hadn't just been ransacking her home . . .'

Valerie felt guilty and uncomfortable that she had to intrude in this way on Ida, but of course she had no choice. To take on this responsibility is to perform a kindness, not commit a violation. Your parents need you to step up and act for them when they can't act for themselves – it's what families are for.

Guide 1 – Selling Their House – How to Talk About It

What not to say

- You won't miss it
- It's much too big for you now – you don't need all that space
- It's getting on top of you – it's in a mess – you can't look after it properly
- You're not coping
- You're too old to look after it
- You'll be able to have a good clear out
- You don't need all this stuff
- You'll be better off without it
- At your age you should be taking it easy

What to say

- It'll be interesting – a new start
- We'll help you find somewhere you'll love
- There's plenty of time to find the right place
- It's time to have some fun – you deserve it
- You'll free up some cash to spend on yourself

At a Glance

- Broach it gently
- Don't rush the process if you can help it
- Keep them informed
- Understand the level of loss
- Where possible, let them *choose*

Chapter 9

DEALING WITH THEIR DEATH

Everyone seems to have a different idea of what death is. Most of us spend our lives studiously ignoring the whole concept, but when we think about it at all, we each interpret it in the way that's most acceptable to us. If we don't believe in any kind of God we can be pragmatic or we can let our imagination – and perhaps an element of wishful thinking – run riot. If we have religious convictions they'll naturally affect our view, but we're still capable of fairly extensive adaptations to accommodate our need to be reassured.

Whatever it turns out to be – a doorway to some kind of heaven, a melding of our atoms with the universe, a journey to a fluffy white cloud, halo and harp, or just final disintegration, death deprives us in *this* life of those we love.

For many of us the first real intimation of this is when our grandparents die. Of course it can be a huge shock, but we're reasonably young when it happens and they seem old by comparison. Our world is rocked, but it readjusts itself and we move on.

The death of a parent is something else again. This time there's no getting away from it – a fundamental part of our existence vanishes. Losing a parent is like the curtain rolling back on the opening scene of a play we don't want to watch;

then when our second parent dies the curtain comes down and we walk out into the cold, alone in a way we've never been before.

It doesn't matter whether you've been close to them or estranged; it makes no difference whether you've loved them or loathed them; their death alters your attitude to your own life in ways you can't anticipate or escape. Whether you're alone or surrounded by loving family, devoted partner and supportive friends, nobody holds your parents' unique place in your life; your roots have just received a brutal hacking.

Suddenly the past is a cul-de-sac. The detailed knowledge of your babyhood, the stories about aunts, uncles and grandparents – the facts and fairytales that make up your image of yourself – have lost their eyewitnesses. The responsibility for your memories now rests with you. The baton has been handed on.

Even if you never really got on with your parents, there *was* a moment when they loved you in a way no one else ever can. It may have been very brief, but it was there. If you've always loved each other, then that love will have enriched your whole life. Either way, without it you'll wobble. Like a table with a leg missing, your balance will suffer.

Then there's the inevitable realization – it's your turn next. The queue has taken a lurch forward and suddenly you're at the head of it. There's nobody now between you and the Grim Reaper. You may be young and fit but you're still the older generation; your status has just changed. It's a sobering thought – enough to account for the slight panic that comes along with everything else you experience when your parents die.

And the death of a parent is unlikely to be completely without baggage. Leaving aside the sadness, there could also be regrets, even guilt; there might be anger, bitterness or resentment within your family. But often there's no need for these feelings; they're a way of sublimating or deflecting your grief. If you can let them go you'll heal faster and feel better about an experience that, one way or another, most of us have to go through.

Facing the Facts

If one of your parents is ill or very frail, then in theory you're expecting the worst. In practice you're probably not accepting the idea at all; as long as they're alive you're likely to be in denial. You know intellectually, but emotionally you can push away the idea, perhaps even lose it in being busy on their behalf. The thing is, your parents are still *there*, just as they've always been.

Sometimes, though, they seem to know better themselves. Josephine's father Leo was in his late seventies.

'My father and I were very close and we saw a lot of each other. One day we were together in his garden and I was helping him prune the roses. We were chatting quietly and out of the blue he said, "If anything happens to me, you won't make me live with your brother will you?" I laughed and said, "Would I?" I knew he'd hate it, because they didn't get on particularly well. Then he said he felt tired and went into the house for a rest.

'Three days later he had a massive stroke, and although he didn't die for several months, he was never able to speak again. I think he'd known something was going to happen.'

It could be simply that Leo felt unwell and it raised questions in his mind that he hadn't considered before. But who knows? There are plenty of examples of what appears to be an uncanny foreknowledge of death.

Marie's mother Lizzie was 85 and still living in her own home.

'Mum had been so well for so long that she used to joke with us about it. She'd tell us she'd still be knitting her charity blanket squares when *our* children were drawing their pension!

'One Saturday I went round for my usual cup of tea and found Mum surrounded by the contents of the bureau. There were papers everywhere, and photos and all kinds of junk.

'I asked her what she was looking for – I thought she'd lost something, but she told me she just thought it was time to sort everything out. She said, "You don't want to have to wade through all this when I'm gone, do you?"

'I brushed it off, but she tried to give me things – a brooch Dad had bought her, a favourite vase. I told her to hang on to them; there was plenty of time yet. There wasn't though – she died a week later. I'm convinced she had a premonition.'

Maybe Lizzie did know she was going to die very soon, maybe not, but Marie wishes she'd accepted those gifts and given Lizzie the pleasure of seeing her with them.

If your parents start behaving in this way it doesn't necessarily mean they know the end is near – they might just have realized in a general way that time will, eventually, run out on them. Don't get maudlin or worry about it. But it will help them if you just take it at face value and accept gracefully without making a fuss.

This realization can take other forms. Queenie is 90 and fairly pragmatic about death. She's made plans about what will happen to her body.

'I told my grandsons I wanted to bequeath my body for medical research. And I'm quite happy to donate my organs – they can have anything they like the look of – it won't be any use to me.

'I've written it all down for after I'm gone, but my grand-sons say, "We know what to do with you, Grandma!"'

Queenie is quite frail but doesn't feel at all sorry for herself. She thinks she might have a few years yet, and she's making the most of them. She's not afraid of the future.

Of course you may know for certain your parent is going to die very soon.

It's a terrible thing to face. But there's another side to this. It gives you all the chance to come to terms with the idea and this can be a very precious opportunity.

Make the most of it. Talk to them, relive old memories, ask those questions you never got around to before; say all the things you'll wish you'd said later; laugh together, say you love each other – say goodbye . . .

Ella's father Daryl was 89 and had been ill for a long time.

'We knew Dad was dying and so did he. The doctors could-n't tell us how long it would be. Dad's always been the straightforward type and he just said we'd live every day for itself and not worry about it. We had some good times and great conversations about everything under the sun.

'I learned more about Dad in those last weeks than I ever had. He told me how he'd courted my mum, stories about the war – things he'd never opened up about before. I wouldn't have missed it. When I remember Dad dying I don't so much think of the misery, I think of all the warmth. It's a *good* memory.'

It might not be easy to do, but clearing the decks emotionally like this will allow the bond between you to become closer and stronger. It will be marvellous for them, and something for you to treasure.

Having a parent seriously ill in hospital is a different thing altogether. It can almost numb you to the idea that they might be going to die soon. Maybe they've been there for months and seen several ups and downs in their condition; perhaps they've been admitted as an emergency and you're reeling from the shock.

The public nature of a hospital can be difficult to handle under these circumstances, even in a side ward or the comparative quiet of intensive care. It might feel impersonal and clinical, but in fact the doctors and nursing staff will be doing everything they can to make the end as peaceful and dignified as possible for your parent and for you. They'll phone you if they think it's going to happen any time soon and tell you what their condition is.

Increasingly these days, when hospitals decide there's nothing more they can do medically, they'll agree to discharge your parent back to their own home, with appropriate professional help, or to their care home (see Chapter 5). This can be an opportunity for you all to have some time and space – a blessing for everyone.

Jonathon's father Wilfred was 93 when he developed a very virulent form of cancer.

'He didn't need prolonged hospital care, so he was able to live in his flat. Social services arranged for hospice nurses to come in every day to give him his pain-killing drugs and treatments. They were wonderful. They don't charge anything, but they're worth their weight in gold. They made Dad's last weeks wonderfully peaceful. I don't know what he'd have done without them.'

Jonathon knows how important it was for his father to spend his last months in his own home, the privacy and dignity this allowed him – and the peace.

Getting through the Crisis

How do you live through something as unimaginable as the death of a parent? You can be in the middle of the crisis before you've had time to grasp it's even happening. Events sweep you along.

But there will be things to give you comfort. Look for the positive – the unexpected kindnesses, love and support from friends, the chance to show your parents how much you care.

When you've been their carer, the sense of loss can be particularly great, but even then there *is* an upside. Juliette's mother Evelyn was 83 and had stomach cancer.

'When Mum became severely ill she went to live with my brother Graham. He put his whole life on hold for her, including his engagement. Mum's illness didn't leave her much dignity but Graham was amazing. He's a hearty, sporty kind of man, and I'd never have expected him to be so gentle. She depended on him for quite intimate things and they coped by making jokes about it. They were very close. The night before she died they were laughing together as he got her into bed.

'Graham took Mum's death really hard. It was months before he recovered, although he did eventually marry his fiancée. She'd been fantastic about the whole thing.'

Evelyn's death altered Graham's life on every level. He didn't just have the loss of his mother to deal with – many of the details of his daily life were swept away at the same time. The routines that had been so vital to his mother's welfare and comfort were suddenly irrelevant; from total responsibility, suddenly there was nothing at all to do for her. It was a fundamental change.

But on the other hand he'd spent his mother's last months drawing close to her in ways he'd never done before. They were painful to live through – of course he grieved. But they left him with good memories and increased respect for her. He was privileged to witness Evelyn's courage and fortitude.

It's possible, though, that if you've been the carer you'll feel relief. Don't be ashamed of this. The responsibility, hard work and general anguish of fulfilling this role make relief absolutely understandable (see Chapter 4). Remember instead how much you've helped your parent, how much you've contributed to their comfort, dignity, happiness and peace of mind.

Sometimes the positive aspects come in another form. Darren's 93-year-old mother Adele had severe Alzheimer's disease and was very frail.

'Mum had been living in her own home with the help of carers but at the end she failed in just a couple of weeks. She fought hard but we all knew it wouldn't be long. It was difficult for us, but it was a huge journey for her doctor too. Their training is to jump on you with electrodes but we'd said we didn't want that to happen.

'Mum's care worker was marvellously understanding. She was very experienced and knew what she was seeing, so when it was getting close she called for us to come. Mum died very peacefully – she just melted away.'

Adele was in a coma and her family was spared the pain of sitting watching her fade unknowingly away, because they trusted her carer to give them time to say goodbye.

The decision families have to make about whether to be there for the end is a very difficult and personal one. You might think you already know what you'll do, but don't be too sure – when it actually happens you might feel quite differently. What do you do, for example, when there's absolutely no chance of your parent waking up and knowing you?

If your parent is unconscious, don't give way to 'sensible' advice about staying away if you feel in your heart that you want to be there. But equally, don't rush off to sit by their bedside and harrow yourself just because you feel you 'should'.

This isn't about anybody else on earth – it's between you and your parent.

Avril's 79-year-old mother Delia had dementia and was living in a care home when she died.

'I sat with Mum for hours. I did *The Times* crossword. People looked askance at me, but she wasn't conscious. The nurse said Mum was asleep and she'd just drift away. She told me it would be soon, so I said a little prayer and left.

'I told myself that if I stayed she might somehow sense what was happening and become worried – she might think "I must be dying". Sometimes your dignity requires that you be in the care of a professional. When your time's coming it's coming, and when you're ready to go, you go. Mum's body had caught up with her mind.

'You hear so often how parents hang on and on, then die as soon as their loved ones are out of the room. It's as though they have to hand over – to die – alone.'

'Mum died in her sleep after I left. I told myself I was leaving because I didn't want to make her afraid, but if I'm honest I wanted a night's sleep too – it was Christmas Eve. It was almost as though I was resentful that she was dying at Christmas.

'It was selfish of me and I feel guilty about it every day. I re-run it, think how it could have been different. I like to do

226

things properly, and I can't get away from the thought that I let myself down.'

Avril is blaming herself for what she did. She loved her mother and made her decision knowing there was nothing else she could do for her, but she was torn two ways. She recognizes that and it worries her.

Yet it was natural to want to get home to make the best Christmas possible under the circumstances for her husband and children. And more than that, doing Christmas things would have made life seem more normal. It would have been touching base with reality, a reality that was nowhere in that room with her mother. Avril should try to forgive herself – if indeed, there's anything to forgive. No one's perfect – we can't live a copybook life.

In fact, deaths that occur at Christmas or on birthdays can be harder to live with in the long term, because everyone else is having a lovely time and there you are, reliving a great sadness. If you avoid the subject it will still be there, hanging over you, more pervasive than ever, so meet it head on.

Try to set aside a special moment for remembering your parents. Make a small ritual of it – after the turkey maybe, or the birthday cake – toast them in their favourite tipple. That's how family traditions are born.

There are circumstances where, whatever the time of year, death can feel like the right thing. Greg's mother Lucille died at 90.

'It happened quite quickly and I was grateful for that. There was less emotional upheaval for her. She'd been missing my dad so badly. It wasn't wrong to be relieved.'

Greg saw clearly what his mother was going through and wanted to see her slide peacefully away. He knows that's what she was wishing for.

Hard as it is to be there when your parents die, it's just as difficult if it happens when you can't be.

Fiona's father Louis was in his seventies.

'We came back from holiday to find a police message telling us to phone Mum at once. Dad had been coping with a blood disorder for a while, but he'd died suddenly and unexpectedly and, though she'd tried, Mum hadn't been able to contact us.

'I couldn't believe it. I'd been very close to my dad and suddenly he wasn't there. The only way to convince myself was to visit his body at the chapel of rest. I'd never have imagined doing this under any circumstances, but it helped me. I looked down at him and thought – that's not my dad. He's really gone then.'

Fiona's father died when her back was turned and seeing his body was her way of bringing it home to herself. But on issues like this make sure you choose what feels right for you. Don't let anyone try to persuade you into their idea of what's appropriate. Do what you feel comfortable with.

Sometimes it can seem your parent is waiting for something; as though, however ill they are, they won't let themselves die until they've witnessed it. This could be the birth of a child, a family wedding, maybe even their own birthday. Then it's almost as if they quietly give permission for death to take them; they've seen what they stayed for – it's all right to go now.

Patrick believes that's what happened to his mother Siobhan.

'When my mother was 89 she had a couple of big strokes. She knew it was almost over and she wasn't well at all, but my granddaughter Rosie's confirmation was coming up and Mum had been looking forward to it for months. She was a very devout lady and it meant a lot to her.

'Mum said, "God will see me right. I think He wants me to stay around for this." Well, He must have done, because we got her into her wheelchair, all dressed up, and she went into that church like a queen.

'She had a ball that day, although it tired her out. She saw all the family, chatted and laughed, even enjoyed some lunch. Rosie was thrilled that her great-granny was there. Mum died just a few days later but that was all right, she'd got what she wanted.'

This was an enormous comfort to Patrick and his family and they smile as they remember that day. Common sense might have dictated that Siobhan wasn't well enough to go – but her heart did, and they knew that, and made it happen.

If one of your parents is faced with waiting for the other to die, you'll need to take on their grief as well as your own, at least at first. You don't have one death to deal with – in some ways you effectively have two.

Kit's wife Pearl died when she was 80.

'We were shopping in a department store and Pearl had gone off on her own to buy a present. I couldn't find her and I just had the feeling that something wasn't right so I asked the store to page her. There was no response.

'Suddenly I saw an ambulance outside and I knew . . .

'I raced out to her. She'd fallen and was unconscious. Her head was bleeding. We never spoke to each other again. I sat by her for three days in the hospital but she never regained consciousness. I tried to talk to her – they say that sometimes your words get through and I was desperate to help. But I don't think she could hear me. She didn't respond. It was just a question of waiting.'

Kit was helped enormously by the presence of his family. At times like this the best thing you can do is simply be there. Take it in turns to spend time with them at the bedside. Help them get some rest if you can, but don't force them into leaving: 'It's for your own good'. If they want to stay it's probably better to let them. Imagine how they – and you – would feel if something happened while they weren't there.

In any case they're likely to be disorientated, confused and unable to come to terms with what's happening. They're suffering from shock and they need you to be strong, whatever you might be going through yourself. And fulfilling that need, focusing on it, can help you through it. In this way the death of a parent can bring families closer together.

But they can be driven apart by it too. The surface of everyday emotions is stripped away and all the insecurities and uncertainties are suddenly exposed. It can be the final straw that splits a fragile relationship.

Colin hadn't always been on the best of terms with his sister Andrea, and it came to a head when their mother Kitty died.

Andrea says:

'Mum had a serious heart attack so I started travelling two hundred miles straight from work every Thursday to spend three days visiting her in hospital, washing her clothes, taking care of her house . . . Colin's own house was close by but he seemed to live at Mum's most of the time. He didn't help. I'd arrive to find the place in a mess and the sink full of his dirty dishes.

'The doctors said that Mum wouldn't be able to manage stairs when she came out of hospital, so I was negotiating with the council to exchange her house for a bungalow, going to look at the options, preparing Mum for the fact that she'd need to move.

'With the worry, travelling and squeezing a demanding full-time job into half the week, I was exhausted and starting to get ill. We'd had a fortnight's holiday booked and my first instinct was to cancel it, but Mum's doctor told me that her recovery would be limited and slow; she could be like that for months. I had to have a rest if I was going to carry on doing this. Colin, of course, said I shouldn't go . . .

'Well, I talked to Mum about it and we went, but the worst happened. She had another heart attack and died in the middle of the holiday. We couldn't get a flight back for a week.

'We got home to find that in just seven days my brother had had Mum cremated, emptied her house and got rid of everything – it was all over.

'Mum had gone and it was like being in a vacuum. Colin accused me of not caring for her at all and we had a truly horrible row. He left me crouching on the floor, completely collapsed with grief and pain.

'We didn't speak for several years, but I've tried a few times to make friends again – after all, he is my brother. I don't think it will ever happen now. I've lost him as well as Mum. It's irrevocable.

'Colin was deeply wrong to behave as he did – it was cruel, unforgivable. But I know that if I had to live through it again, this time I wouldn't leave her. I'd listen to my instinct.'

Andrea feels she deserted her mother when she needed her most, but in fact she'd been there – and was still there – for her. She couldn't have known what was going to happen; even the doctors got it wrong. Only hindsight has 20/20 vision.

Andrea's experience shows how hard it can be to divorce your own needs from what your love for your parents, or what you feel is your duty, is telling you to do. And someone will almost always find something to criticize; it's easy to be wise when you're a third party. There's no simple answer of course. You have to work it out for yourself.

You can only do your best, but that's enough – your parents would expect no more.

Colin was probably feeling anger and frustration as well as grief at losing his mother. He lashed out at the nearest person – his sister – and their relationship has been destroyed. It's the very last thing any mother would want. If you find yourself at odds with your family at a time like this, try to hold back, if only for your parents' sake.

Serena's mother Jeanine had been incapacitated by a massive stroke and was in hospital.

'The hospital told my brother Oliver that Mum had become seriously unwell, but he didn't let me know. She died while I was out playing golf. When I confronted Oliver he said he'd wanted to spare me. I was angry because poor Mum was on her own when she died. If I'd known I'd have gone to her. I didn't fall out with Oliver, but I have wondered since why he did it.'

Serena and her mother were very close, and it's possible Oliver felt jealous of their relationship. Of course he might have been telling the truth about wanting to spare her – or it could have been a mixture of the two he himself couldn't entirely fathom.

Losing someone you love can produce a tangle of emotions. Feelings can surface you didn't even know you had and your own jealousies and resentments can take you by surprise. Don't let them rip if you can help it. They might have some basis in reality, but they're often exacerbated by grief.

What to Do Next

The loss of a parent is such a big shock it can incapacitate you. The bottom drops out of your world and you go into free fall.

What do you do next? You may never have had to deal with the formalities of a death before and, unlike a wedding, they're not something people tend to chat about. The practicalities aren't very complex, but there are routines to be gone through. They can vary regionally, and some of them are mandatory.

If your parent has died after an illness and has been seen by the doctor within the last fourteen days the procedure is straightforward. If the death was at home their GP will need to be called in to determine the cause of death and issue a certificate. You then take this, along with their birth certificate and medical card if you have it, to your parent's local Registrar's Office to register the death. They'll give you a certificate for burial or cremation. An undertaker can't proceed without this.

If it happened in hospital, the staff will put you in touch with the bereavement officer, who will arrange for a death certificate and tell you to talk to your parent's GP.

On the other hand, if the doctor hasn't seen your parent for a while and doesn't know why they died, the case is referred to the coroner's office to arrange a postmortem to determine the cause of death. This will usually take place very quickly.

When the death is found to be from natural causes, the death certificate is issued. If it's found to be sudden death – say an accident or a fall – the coroner may call an inquest, but this won't necessarily slow down the funeral because the coroner can issue an interim certificate.

Nat's mother Cora died in her care home.

'I had a call to say that Mum had fallen out of bed and cut her face. The care home had sent her to hospital for some stitches but she was otherwise OK. Twenty-four hours later the doctor told us that she was deeply unconscious and bleeding into her brain. He said she wouldn't recover.

'The hospital sent Mum back to her care home, which we

were very glad about. She died there a few days later but a death certificate couldn't be issued because it wasn't clear whether the bleeding was from natural causes or had been brought on by the fall.

'They did a postmortem the following day, which showed that she'd died of a stroke that had nothing to do with the fall, so the doctor was able to sign the death certificate. If they'd found that the fall had caused her death, there would have been an inquest.'

Organizing a funeral

Most people contact a funeral director to act for them. They'll move the body, liaise with the coroner's office if necessary, arrange a coffin, book the crematorium if appropriate, and take on a lot of the paperwork and organization for you.

It's best to get a few quotes beforehand. Ask firms to spell out what the charges cover. And check whether your parents have taken out a pre-paid funeral plan. It's quite common for elderly people to do this.

The biggest decisions can be whether to have a burial or cremation, whether or not to have a religious service and if so what form it should take, and where your parents will be laid to rest – a church graveyard or a municipal cemetery, for example. But all cultures and religions have their own habits, customs and rules.

If your parents have expressed strong wishes or left instructions about this, your job is easy – you can follow them. If they've had a religious faith that simplifies things too – you can talk to their vicar/priest/church leader and get all the guidance you need on how to proceed. Your parents may even have already bought a plot for burial, or there may be a family grave to be opened up.

You should check if your parent has left any instructions about giving their body for medical research or donating their organs. They could even have written an advance directive about it (see Chapter 7).

If you have a surviving parent, listen to them. However strong your own convictions may be, religious or otherwise, a major part of the job of this funeral has to be to help *them*. But if nothing has ever been said, you have the knotty problem of guessing what they'd have wanted and marrying that with what you and the rest of the family feel should happen (see Chapter 1).

Glenys and Ivor are in their eighties and had never talked about funerals until recently.

Ivor says:

'We should talk about it now, though – after all, it isn't getting further away is it? Glenys has written down some hymns and probably I ought to do the same. I've sung in the church choir all my life but I don't want a church funeral. I'd rather have a memorial service later when everyone can have a smile and a good sing.

'We had thought of arranging for one of those pre-paid funerals, but then we decided to spend the money on a walk-in shower instead. It would be helpful for Glenys's arthritis and it would give us a project. You have to think positive.'

It's a good job Ivor is telling his family his wishes now, because it's a pretty safe bet that, knowing his Christian beliefs, they'd have given him a church service.

Wherever they're held and whatever form they take, funerals can be an important emotional milestone. They're a chance to celebrate your parents' life; to let go, weep unrestrainedly and unashamedly together with a lot of people who loved your parents too. It's a rite of passage for all of you and it can help you to grieve and get over it.

Della's mother Marigold was 90 when she died.

'All Mum's great-grandchildren were at her funeral. They'd written letters to her and tied them to helium balloons. It was a wonderful moment when they let them float up into the sky. We had her ashes scattered in the garden of rest at the crematorium and my little grandson said, "Granny's in the most beautiful garden in the world, isn't she?"'

Not everyone believes children should be present at funerals, and this is one of those subjects that can cause arguments in families. The decision depends on so many factors – the age and personality of the child and whether *they* want to go, the way they've been brought up, how close they were to your parent, and the kind of funeral you'll be holding.

When 85-year-old Ethel died, her granddaughter Chloe took her baby daughter Annette to the funeral. Chloe's mother Angie was pleased.

'Annette was only eighteen months old – far too young to be upset by what was going on, but she transformed the day for everyone else. She was like a ray of sunshine – she cheered us all up. And it was especially wonderful for my husband, who was saying goodbye to his mum, to have her there.

'I can't help thinking it was a symbol of continuity. The very youngest member of the family was smiling at everyone as we said goodbye to the oldest. It was like shouting – "Life goes on, feel good about it!"'

What do you do after the funeral? The custom has grown up to have some kind of refreshment, simply because people often have to travel a long way to be there. But there's no rule about it. If you prefer, everyone can just drive away.

Some families have huge parties; the Jewish custom is to sit shivah for several days, with family and friends constantly coming in and out, bringing food, love and support; Irish tradition is to hold a wake, where alcohol – and emotion – can flow freely.

A get-together can be a good way of leaving the day on an upbeat note. Thomas's family do this.

'When there's a funeral in our family we always have a party, and so when Mum died we booked a buffet lunch at the local pub, put some cash behind the bar, and everybody came.

'They all arrived from the church looking sad and solemn, but in a few minutes they were chatting about Mum, reminiscing, laughing. It's great because we have a big family and the only time they all get together is at weddings and funerals.'

This kind of tradition helps keep the family functioning as a unit, and breaks the ice, helping you to start talking straight away about the person you've lost.

Try to work it all out between you – hymns, flowers, get-together. Whatever you choose to do, high profile or quiet and private, you want to be able to look back afterwards and think – Mum (or Dad) would have enjoyed that. It was a good sendoff.

Dealing with probate

Probate is the legal procedure that enables the money and property in your parent's estate to be released to whomever is to inherit it. The details vary regionally. England and Wales are the same but Scotland and Northern Ireland may have differences, so you need to check with the Probate Registry where your parents were living.

One person (sometimes more than one) is given the legal right – a 'Grant' – to gather together everything your parent has to leave, pay outstanding debts and then give out the rest according to the will, or, if there is no will, according to the law.

The person who does this has usually been named as an executor in the will, but if no one has been appointed or a will doesn't exist, then it can be carried out by whoever is the next of kin (there's an order of priority). Either way you have to apply to the Probate Office for a Grant of Representation. There are some circumstances where a Grant might not be required – perhaps if the estate is very small. Again, you need to check this.

To apply for a Grant you'll have to fill in forms and attend an interview at which you'll be asked to swear an oath or sign a document stating that the information you've given is correct.

Once probate has been granted, you'll be able to obtain the release of your parent's funds from banks, building societies and so on, to pay their debts. Then you're legally obliged to disburse the rest to whoever is entitled to it.

If the estate is a simple one you can do all this yourself, but most people consult a solicitor.

Helping a Surviving Parent

Difficult though it is for you to face a world without one of your parents, it's much, much harder for the parent who's left behind. Think about it – think how empty life must seem.

The person who knew you best, cared about you most and remembered you in your prime, is gone. That's a very lonely feeling.

And if one of your parents has been caring for the other through their last illness, the loss will be a double blow.

When Kelly's mother Becky died, her father Bernard seemed to age.

'Dad had been very healthy – he'd been taking the strain of Mum's care for about a year, and even though we knew that her cancer was terminal, he'd been positive, cheery, a real tonic to Mum and to us. He did everything for her. Then when she died he just went to half-volume. He looked ten years older and started acting it too.

'I took him to the pub one lunchtime and asked him about it. He told me that with Mum gone, he was *bored*. Suddenly he had all this time on his hands and it gave him the chance to think about death – not just hers, his own. Dad said growing old wasn't so bad when you had someone to do it with, but it was pretty scary on your own.

'I look after my grandchildren on Friday teatimes and I asked Dad if he'd like to come over every week and give me a hand. He jumped at it. He'd missed out on getting to know them properly because the kids would have disturbed Mum too much, and Dad could never leave her for long. Now he's really close to them – they think the world of him. It's fantastic for all of them. Mum would have been pleased.'

Bernard's life could have become a blank space. Instead it gave him new people to love. Tragically, this kind of resolution isn't always possible.

Wayne's mother Danielle was 82 when his father Claude died.

'Mum had Alzheimer's disease, and sometimes she was

lucid, sometimes not so much so. When Dad died she didn't seem to take it in, and she'd wander round, saying, "I'm just going to look for your dad." Every time we told her Dad was dead there was a fresh wash of grief, as if she was hearing it for the first time. In a way she was . . .

'To spare Mum, we stopped trying to make her aware of Dad's death. When she asked where he was, we'd just say he was in another room, or making a cup of tea.'

For Wayne and his family, it seemed kinder to do this than keep putting Danielle through this fearful time warp.

Desperate grief isn't confined to people in Danielle's situation. Rosemary's mother Ivy was widowed at 71.

'Mum and Dad were devoted to each other and his death completely overthrew her. She'd been visiting him at all hours in the hospital, and then he died one day after she'd left. It horrified her that she hadn't said goodbye. She agonized about whether to see him in the chapel of rest but the thought was just too awful for her and in the end she didn't go.

'When the hearse drew up to the house on the day of the funeral, Mum just fell to pieces. She rushed upstairs and wouldn't come down. We calmed her sufficiently to go through with it, but that was effectively the end of the mum we knew.

'She changed completely. Mum had been *young* – full of life, gregarious, chatty. When Dad died she became withdrawn, bitter, bad-tempered. She just gave up.'

'We tried to break her out of it. We told her that Dad had worshipped her and would never have wanted her to be so unhappy; that she had years of good life ahead of her; that we loved her, her grandchildren loved her. It made no difference – she didn't really want to live a day after Dad went. She died two years later from a heart attack. I don't think she'd had a truly happy moment in all that time.'

Losing her husband took away Ivy's appetite for life. She knew she had a loving family to live for, but they weren't enough, which was a sad realization for them. They did their best to keep her attached to life, but in the end the pain was too much to bear.

Although everyone reacts differently, grief does tend to follow a pattern. At first your parent might not be able to believe that it's really happened. Then, when they do accept it, they could go through several stages of anger, bitterness, even fear at the thought of coping on their own for the first time in maybe half a century. Try to explain that it's natural for them to feel like this, that gradually they'll regain their confidence and balance and be able to take up the threads of life again.

Of course, the death of one of your parents can leave the other unable to cope alone and they may need to move into a care home or sheltered accommodation. This means they'll be losing two things at once and you'll need to handle them very gently indeed (see Chapter 4).

Even if they're well enough to live alone, having your surviving parent to stay with you for a while can work wonders, and help bring them back into the real world. A break like this will give them new scenes, new routines, something else to think about – a fresh perspective. Being with people they love can be a tremendous boost.

But it can be risky too, if they've come straight to you after their partner has died, and never slept at home since. The emotional build-up to going home to an empty house, the place, perhaps, where their partner actually died, can be completely daunting. They might well be terrified at the idea of even walking through the door, let alone going back there to live. Who can blame them?

Going home, they'll have to face their loss squarely, something they might have been able to avoid while staying with you. As they walk through the rooms they shared, as the everyday things around them bring their life together into sharp focus, they'll feel the full impact of their situation and the loneliness that awaits them. And the longer they stay with you, the harder it will be to step back into reality.

While they're with you, talk about 'when you go home' as a positive thing, as inevitable, something that's understood between you. Don't make a big deal of it, but understand that it will be for them. Mention it briefly right from the start, but don't be dismissive if the prospect frightens them.

Try to build up their confidence gradually. You could help reintroduce their hobbies while they're with you. If they live near enough, invite their friends to visit. Contact fellow churchgoers or club members and ask them to stay in touch too.

It can be helpful to make some brief trips to break the ice before they actually move back properly. You could spend a few short sessions sorting out their partner's clothes together, for example. They'll need your help and support in this, and if it's feasible it can be better to do it in small bites than one exhausting visit. And later it might also help to ease the final transition if you spend the first couple of nights there with them, just to settle them in.

Having your parent with you will also give you the chance to keep an eye on their health. The effects of grief can be far-reaching – they might not be eating much or sleeping very well and this can leave them without the energy or spirits to fight their way back to life.

But a visit like this can be tricky for *you*. When Tess's

father Walter died after a severe stroke, his wife Leonora was heartbroken.

'Dad was very ill for some time and it destroyed my mother. She wasn't emotionally capable of coping with it. She just walked the boards and cried. When he died Mum was so upset she couldn't go to the funeral.

'She came to stay with us straight away and just gave herself up to grief. She'd sit rubbing her hankie and crying all the time. One day I lost it and shouted at her. I know I shouldn't have, but I was worn out, I couldn't help myself. Mum was grieving, but so was I. We never referred to it again, and soon after that she went to stay with my sister.

'Later she moved into a new flat and seemed happier, but she never talked about my father at all. Yet they'd been together for sixty years; they were terribly close.'

Leonora couldn't handle the reality of her husband's death, and Tess was having trouble dealing with it too. Soothing someone who needs constant attention and support is tiring, emotionally and physically, and watching her mother suffering so much brought her own grief home to her more forcibly.

If you find yourself getting irritated, try hard not to show it. Sometimes it can take virtual sainthood to bite your lip, but you'll be glad you did. Remember what they're going through. Don't give yourself regrets you'd rather spend the rest of your life without.

Everyone finds their own way of dealing with grief. It can seem easier if, like Leonora, you never refer to the person you've lost. That way you won't have to feel the pain, you won't risk being moved to tears. But it's not really helping at all. You're effectively in denial, bottling everything up and pretending you're fine.

Howard's parents Henrietta and Giles were both 80 and living in a care home.

'When Dad died Mum was very upset. She cried at the funeral, but then she never mentioned Dad again. We'd bring him into the conversation but she'd just ignore it.

'I did wonder if Mum was half glad Dad was gone. Don't get me wrong, she loved him. But she'd looked after him for a long time and it had made her ill. It would have been natural for her to feel relieved that the burden had finally been lifted – none of us would have blamed her.'

But Henrietta might have blamed herself. And she'd have felt very guilty about it, wondering how she could be even slightly glad that her husband of sixty years had died. She wouldn't have been able to face the thought, and refusing to discuss him was her solution.

In fact, she finally did start talking about Giles in the few weeks before she herself died. She'd come to terms with it at last.

If your parent won't discuss their loss, persevere. Just hearing the sound of his or her name will be good for them. Chat between yourselves when they're in the room. They'll listen even if they don't join in, and gradually they might be able to bring up the subject themselves.

The more you steer clear of it, the harder it will be to broach, until it becomes a no-go area – a tragedy for them, because the greater part of their past life will just disappear.

Jeannie isn't in any doubt that her mother Cora was relieved when her father Joshua died, although they've never discussed it.

'To be truthful, I think Mum had been looking forward to it. Dad had changed, you see. He wouldn't go on holidays or join in anything and she'd get cross and nag him about it. We discovered later that he'd been ill for a long time before anyone realized it. I think Mum must have known deep down that it was illness that was causing him to be miserable. But she never admitted it afterwards.'

Perhaps Cora had found it easier to put Joshua's changed personality down to plain grumpiness than to face the fact that he might be ill. Grumpiness you can tackle – illness is more frightening altogether.

Reluctance to face facts can take all kinds of forms. Adam's father Alastair died at 73.

'We'd all known that Dad's illness was terminal, but he never talked about it. He was always cheerful; his way was just to ignore it and carry on as though everything was normal. That meant we all had to do the same, and made it very hard for Mum when he died because they hadn't come to terms with it at all.

'Dad had written a diary all his life, right through the war and ever since. We knew it existed but we'd never seen it. After he died I asked Mum if we could read it, but she'd burned it.

'Dad had written in his diary all the things he found impossible to say aloud about his illness and impending death. Mum said it had been so heartbreaking, so personal, that she could never have let us see it. She'd destroyed it to protect him.'

'I absolutely respect her instinct but I wish she'd kept the diaries from before his illness. Those books would have been a fantastic record of Dad's life – something for us to hand down to the great-grandchildren he never knew in person.

'Looking back I wonder if I'd tried harder I could have got

Dad to talk to me about his fears and feelings. I wish he hadn't felt he needed to go through it alone. He was such a private person.'

Adam feels he let his father down because Alastair didn't confide in him; that somehow he fell short. But everyone has compulsions and inner drives. Alastair couldn't suddenly become demonstrative after a lifetime of diffidence.

Adam needs to understand that his father loved them all, and was probably trying to find a way to spare them pain.

As Time Goes By

In the aftermath of their loss a surviving parent is going to need you to tell them there's still something worth living for – that they still *matter.* Your life takes on a different shape when you lose your partner – meals, chores, what you watch on TV and so on. Your daily routine changes to accommodate one, not two. It can seem as though it's hardly worth getting up in the morning. Why cook, why clean – why bother?

If you haven't been on your own before it's hard to have no backup. You were part of a team, now you're solo. And it's more than that; it can seem you've lost your validation, you're no longer important to anyone in the same way you were to your partner – you have no role; your family might love you a lot but nobody actually *needs* you any more.

Even if you live in a community where everyone knows you, this can leave you feeling very isolated. Verity remembers how her mother behaved after she was widowed.

'Mum had always loved having people to talk to, and looking back I think she was very lonely on her own. She didn't give up on life, but you could tell she was frustrated. I saw a lot of her but I wish now I'd asked her if there was anything she specially wanted to do. I didn't think of it.'

It's tempting to think that once a bereaved person has had a year or so to get over it they won't need any special help – but that's just when they need it most. The fuss is over and everything has gone back to normal – except that for them nothing will ever be normal again.

Harris is 87, and lost his wife Mabel four years ago.

'I was surrounded by my family. That was wonderful. It took my mind off things.

'And Mabel had so many friends. Even now they still come up to me in the street and give me a hug or a kiss – and I don't even know their names! It's fantastic. In a way she's still supporting me, even though she's gone.

'But there's a huge hole in my life. I'm dreadfully lonely. My life's getting emptier and emptier – the visitors seem to have dried up. You wonder what you've done to make them drop you. I can't cook so I don't feel I can invite anyone round. And Mabel was such good company. I need someone to talk to.

'I find myself talking all sorts of rubbish to all sorts of strange people, babbling about my bad back and so on. I wouldn't do it if Mabel were here. I put on a brave face but I'm very depressed – in fact I'm terrified of depression.'

Harris is missing the shorthand of married life. The ability to chat on any and every subject just as it arises, without the need for explanations or excuses. It's rather like having your microphone switched off – you're talking but no one can hear you.

If your parent isn't coping further down the line, ask the doctor to drop by for a chat. They may just be feeling sad, and it can help having someone professional to talk to. On the other hand they may be suffering from clinical depression. This is a treatable illness and the doctor will know what to look for.

Even if you live a long way from your surviving parent, try to visit as often as you can. It's vital to do this and to keep on doing it when the first shock wears off.

Even if your parent seems to be coping well, they'll need you to be there for them. They'll still have ups and downs, good weeks and bad weeks. Lots of company and things to interest them will keep them positive.

When Hywel's wife Bronwen died several years ago, his ten-year-old granddaughter Callie had a plan.

'Callie started sending me little letters every couple of weeks – the most beautiful wording, decorated with stickers and with SWALK on the envelope. She still does it. They're wonderful.'

This kind of loving thoughtfulness is exactly what's needed to keep the demons at bay. If there are children in your family get them together and suggest they do something similar. They could take it in turns. Explain how sad it is always to be missing someone. Young children in particular have a huge fund of compassion, tenderness and imagination – it only needs tapping.

It can be tempting to suggest that your parent moves house to get away from the memories (see Chapter 8), but you need to gauge their state of mind carefully. Some will find comfort in the tangible presence of their partner's things, while it might make others grieve even harder.

Leonie's parents Olivia and Rupert were still living in their own house, and she tried to persuade them to downscale to something more manageable.

'They wouldn't move out of their home, but then Dad died and Mum agreed to sell the house. Looking back I'm glad it worked out this way. She had a fresh start. If I'd managed to move them before he died, now she'd have to

live with all those painful reminders and sit looking at his empty chair.'

Leonie knew Olivia would find it hard to cope surrounded by reminders of Rupert. She realized, too, that a new project would appeal to her mother, and take her mind off her loneliness. A clean break might be hard to face at first, but it can work wonders.

When Lee's father Dominic died, his mother Mirabelle was 80.

'After Dad's death Mum upped sticks and whizzed off on her own to start a new life in a new place. She began to paint and to our amazement she was as good as Dad, who'd been a professional commercial artist. We hadn't known she had this talent, but she said, "Well, of course, your dad and I met at art school." When they got married she'd put all her training aside to be a wife and mother. That's what women did – they gave up things.

'Mum's 96 now and has had to stop painting, although she's still alert enough to do the crossword. She coped with Dad's death, got over it, even though they were so close they shut out other people.'

Mirabelle was typical of her generation; a wife's life was often subsumed in that of her husband. She hadn't resented – or even questioned – giving up her art. Dominic's death freed her to indulge her talent for the first time.

Moving On

It's natural to try to rationalize what you're going through when your parents die. If they had a long illness you might console yourself with the thought that they wanted to die, that they were ready – and it might well be true. Or if the death was sudden, you might tell yourself they'd had a long and happy life; that this is the way they'd have preferred to go, no lingering pain or fear, just here one minute, gone the next – and this might be true too. If your parent was missing their partner, you could convince yourself they wanted to be together.

Positive thinking can be very comforting. It's all part of the mechanism that helps us cope with tragedy. Once again the human survival instinct keeps our head above water.

But we also have a substantial capacity for hindsight, and therefore guilt. When we look back on the last years of their lives, it's natural to have some regrets, even if they're only mild ones. It's probably always possible to think 'I could have done that better'.

Gary's father Luke died in his late seventies.

'My dad had had several strokes and they'd left him deaf. It wasn't treatable and he couldn't communicate very well. He was too old to learn to lip-read so he'd write things down, but muddle them.

'It all tended to exclude him from what was going on around him – he couldn't keep up; he'd miss things and get cross about it. The frustration made him almost bitter.

'Looking back, I wish I'd understood – really understood – what it must have felt like to be unable to take part in so much of normal life. He must have known I loved him, but I feel I could have shown him more affection and given him more support. I would have found ways to do it if I'd tried. It just didn't occur to me.'

Gary isn't eaten up with unreasonable regret and guilt, but he sees clearly from a distance what he was too close to see before.

For your parents' sake and your own peace of mind, it's worth taking an objective look now at what's going on in their lives, making an imaginative journey into what it's like to be them and asking yourself whether there's anything you can do or say, organize or facilitate, to make their lives more fun, reduce their frustration, show them you understand and care.

This is particularly important if only one of them is still living. Lance's mother Vivienne died at 83.

'Mum had always wanted to see Paris – for some reason she and my father had never gone there. After he died I said I'd take her, but she became too ill to go before we got around to it. It wasn't anyone's fault, she was busy and so were we, but it's a shame she missed it. I'd like to think I'd given her that before it was too late.'

If you have any plans, try not to put them off. Don't tell yourself they'll tire your parents too much, or that there's plenty of time when they're stronger or fitter. You never know what's around the corner.

Once we've gone through the trauma of losing our parents we should, in theory, have a relatively anxiety-free period before *we* get too old; when we can, for possibly the first time since we were young, truly live for ourselves and have some fun.

Because everyone's living so much longer, the period between our parents' deaths and our own old age is actually getting shorter. That makes it important to come to terms with it, let that survival instinct have its way and move on.

Otherwise we can squander our chance for a last fling by anticipating our own demise. Of course we'll miss our parents, but we should be able to look back with pleasure, feel that

251

they're still with us, they've never really left. If we can do that, death will have lost at least some of its sting.

The way we remember them is key to this. Family memories are vital – they give us a past and help to forge our future.

When Roddy's father Basil died, his mother gave him the diaries Basil had written during the war and in the early years of his marriage.

'Mum and Dad had been in the army together and it was fascinating to read about their work, the weekend passes when they went dancing, how they missed each other when they were posted apart.

'The diary went through their wedding and demobilization, their first home, a miscarriage, my birth. Through Dad's eyes I saw my parents as they'd been when they were young, with the same hopes, fears and plans that we all have. The diaries stopped with Dad getting the job he wanted. He wrote "everything looks rosy". They were all set for a happy life.'

And it did have a happy ending. Roddy's parents had sixty years together. They weren't rich, but they didn't need to be. They were fulfilled.

Roddy's mother is dead now too, but that diary is a line into his parents' past, *their* time, keeping his thoughts of them alive.

If your parents were ill for a long time, or had dementia, it can be difficult to get past the image of them like that and think back to how they used to be when they were *themselves*.

Karen's father-in-law Jeremy had Alzheimer's disease and died at 85.

'Jeremy's Alzheimer's had been slowly developing for a few years, and by the end his personality was pretty far gone.

I was looking through some of his papers after he died and found something he'd written for the parish magazine before he was ill.

'I read this clever, funny piece reflecting on the changes he'd seen in a long life and it moved me to tears. Suddenly there he was in front of me – a vibrant, jolly man who loved dancing and package holidays – a great swimmer, fit, never happier than when he was sitting in the sun in shorts, topless and with a beer in his hand. I remembered his brown torso, his big laugh, his jokes, how he teased his grandchildren.

'I'd known him since I was sixteen – a wonderfully kind man who bought me a winter coat when I was too poor as a student to afford one. How could I have forgotten the way he'd flirted with me (harmlessly) for over forty years? How could I have replaced his huge, confident personality with a grey shadow?

'Finding that piece of paper brought Jeremy back to life for me, and I'll remember him now the way he lived, not how he died.'

It's very easy to 'lose' your parents in this way, and get stuck with a picture of pale old age – great infirmity, great pain. And if their personality changed over their last weeks or months – even years – under the strains of growing old, it's fatally easy to remember them like that too – bitter, angry and fearful (see Chapter 3).

But you will get round this. Gradually, over time, you'll find flashes of the real person – the person you knew for most of your life – coming back to you. There are plenty of ways to help this happen.

Owen's mother Addy died in her eighties.

'My sisters and I were all left some cash. I could have used it for something mundane like repairing dents on the car

or just put it into the bank, but I felt it was more important than that. It's an emotional thing. I wanted to use it to pay for something special so I built a new garden. It's a daily reminder of my mother.'

Addy probably wouldn't have minded what Owen had used the money for – she'd no doubt have been glad it came in handy for any purpose – but Owen did what felt right to him, and it comforts him and keeps his mother in the front of his mind.

You could donate a park bench, or pay for the church to be floodlit one night a year, or simply plant a tree in your garden – anything that seems appropriate to their lives and yours.

It's important, because whatever afterlife awaits us (always supposing one awaits us at all), our immortality in *this* life is in the memories of the people we leave behind. So talk to each other about your parents, think about them. Don't let them fade away.

Corinne's maternal grandfather died when she was three.

'I can just about remember sitting on Granddad Dudley's knee. I have a mental image of a big man, a large grey waist-coat and a moustache, but I was too young for other memories to stick.

'Mum used to tell us a wonderful story about him. Granddad was a publican and he had a customer called Arthur who loved to moan. He'd stand at the bar month after month saying life wasn't worth living, that he'd kill himself, until Granddad got fed up with it. He said, "If you really want to do it, I'll cut your throat for you if you like," and told him to come the next day.

'When Arthur arrived he looked around nervously and saw a collection of big vicious-looking butchers' knives in a bowl, but Granddad sat him down in a big chair, draped towels round his neck and told him not to worry, if he closed his eyes and put his head back he wouldn't feel a thing. Arthur did as he was told.

'Granddad dipped the largest of the knives in a bucket of boiling water and ran the back of the scalding blade across Arthur's throat, saying, "That'll teach you!"

'Arthur leapt out of the chair and ran down the road screaming, "He's killed me, the blighter's killed me!"

'As Mum said – he never moaned again.'

That story brings Dudley to life as the great practical joker he was. It adds a third dimension to the faded black-and-white photographs in the family shoebox. Corinne will tell it to her grandchildren and it will continue to be told for generations beyond anyone who ever knew Dudley. It's a legend.

Your stories don't need to be dramatic. Little everyday tales will work the same magic, pulling your parents back from the past, lighting them up in the present.

The beauty of storytelling is that it enables you to smile at their faults as well as their finer points. So do it with tolerance and understanding. You don't need to lie, but be kind to their memory, just as you hope one day your children will be kind to yours.

If your parents are still alive, ask them to tell you stories from their own past and from when *their* parents were young. You'll treasure them later. When your parents do die, start passing on stories straight away, while the people who lived in them are still fresh in your mind. If you all got on well there will be plenty of material. Even if you didn't, think hard. You'll still find something worth telling.

Don't get yourself stuck in a loop reliving things you wish were different, blaming yourself – or them – for things you can never change. Let it go and remember the good stuff.

Birthday parties, hilarious Christmases, disasters like rained-off camping holidays and the time you all spent New Year's Eve with a tummy bug and a glass of water – they're all grist to the mill.

If you have grandchildren you're in luck – you've got a ready-made audience. They'll lap it up. You can tell them endless tales and they'll keep coming back for more – and for their favourite ones over and over again.

Sit your grandchildren down on a rainy day and instead of yet another re-run of *The Little Mermaid* or *Harry Potter*, entertain them with tales of the 'olden days'.

So much has happened in the last century, including two world wars and the moon landings; so many things have changed – we've gone from clogs and outside privies to trainers and en-suite bathrooms, from horse-drawn carts to supercars, from magic lanterns to computers.

Whether they're four or fourteen there will be fascinating things you can tell your grandchildren. Get out that shoebox and talk them through it. It's social history; it's real, it's *your* history – and that makes it theirs too.

Sing them the songs that were sung to you when you were small. Keep the continuity – pass it down. Teach them to love your parents in retrospect and *you'll* love them more too.

It's a win/win situation.

Guide 1 – After the Death

Paperwork	What it does
Death Certificate Gives cause of death. Issued by GP (or hospital doctor) immediately in the case of natural death (e.g. when they've seen your parent within 14 days). If death is sudden – e.g. doctor hasn't visited for some time – a post mortem may be required to determine cause of death. This will take place very quickly. If it's found to be due to natural causes, then issued as above. If it was caused by an accident, fall etc. then there may need to be an inquest. Coroner will normally issue an interim certificate so the funeral can proceed.	Enables you to register your parent's death. Take the death certificate, plus your parent's birth certificate and medical card to their local Registrar's office (see local phone book). You'll need copies of the death certificate for probate.
Certificate for burial or cremation.	Issued at registration of death by the Registrar to enable burial or cremation to take place. Funeral director can't act without it.
Social Security Form	May be issued as above by the Registrar for any arrears due to the person who has died and to enable widow/widower to claim benefits.

Guide 2 – Probate

Grant of representation	Contact
Issued by the probate registry, enabling the holder to access and release the money and goods in the estate.	Probate Helpline 0845 3020900 for local addresses Northern Ireland: Probate and Matrimonial Office 02890 724679 Citizens' Advice Bureaux (see local phone book). Age Concern has fact sheets and information on local procedure Age Concern England 0800 009966 www.ace.org.uk Northern Ireland 02890 325055 www.ageconernni.org Scotland 0845 1259732 www.ageconcernscotland.org.uk Cymru 02920 431555 www.accymru.org.uk

Guide 3 – Arranging a Funeral

What to Do	Who Can Help
Get estimates from funeral directors. Check what their costs include.	The National Association of Funeral Directors has a code of practice: 0845 2301343 www.nafd.org.uk Citizen's Advice Bureaux (see local phone book)
For a church funeral – you can have this even if your parent is being cremated. Discuss hymns, music, readings, eulogy.	Contact the church or get the funeral director to do it
For a burial – either ashes or body. Will there be room in the graveyard? Is there a family plot? Have your parents bought ground in a cemetery?	Contact the church
For a cremation – do you want a religious service? Music? Organist and hymns? Will you want the ashes scattered or buried at the crematorium?	Talk to your funeral director The Cremation Society of Great Britain has advice 01622 688292 www.cremation.org.uk
For a non-religious funeral	British Humanist Association 020 7079 3580 www.humanism.org.uk National Secular Society Advice, forms of words 020 7404 3126 www.secularism.org.uk
Make your own arrangements	Natural Death Centre 0871 2882098 www.naturaldeath.org.uk Advice on arranging DIY funerals
Put notices in the local papers to inform people of the funeral time and place, or simply to announce the death.	Phone local newspapers

Guide 4 – Dealing with Bereavement

Useful Contacts	What They Do
Age Concern Local phone number or national numbers in Guide 2	May offer bereavement counselling
Cruse Bereavement Care Helpline: 0870 1671677 www.crusebereavement- care.org.uk	Offers support, counselling, information leaflets
The Compassionate Friends 0845 1232304 www.tcf.org.uk	Offers support for the bereaved and their families.
Samaritans 0845 7909090	24-hour helpline

At a Glance

- Come to terms with it together
- Do your best and don't feel guilty
- Understand what a surviving parent is going through
- Don't fight with your family
- Remember your parents at their best
- Keep family stories alive

INDEX